Mini-Invasive Surgery of the Hip

Dominique G. Poitout • Henri Judet

Editors

Mini-Invasive Surgery
of the Hip

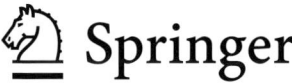 Springer

Editors

Dominique G. Poitout
Professeur des Universités
Service de chirurgie et de traumatologie
CHU de Marseille – Hôpital Nord
Marseille
France

Henri Judet
Service de Chirurgie Orthopédique et
Traumatologie
Clinique Jouvenet
Paris
France

Additional material to this book can be downloaded from http://extras.springer.com.

ISBN 978-2-287-79930-3   ISBN 978-2-287-79931-0   (eBook)
DOI 10.1007/978-2-287-79931-0
Springer Paris Heidelberg New York Dordrecht London

Library of Congress Control Number: 2014935369

Printed on acid-free paper

Springer is part of Springer Science+Business Media (www.springer.com)

Extra Materials on http://extras.springer.com

Contents

Chapter 1
Minimally Invasive Anterior Approach for Total Hip Replacement

Thierry Siguier, Marc Siguier, and Bertrand Brumpt

Abstract The minimally invasive anterior approach using intermuscular planes allows a surgical approach to the hip and implantation of a total hip prosthesis with no muscle, tendon, or trochanteric section, even partially. This is not offered by any other surgical approach. Preserving the abductors and gluteal muscles with an approach that is distant to them avoids the risk of limp attributable to insufficiency of the gluteus medius. The minimally invasive anterior approach for THR is a safe and reproducible technique providing low morbidity and fast postoperative recovery.

Introduction

The most widely used approaches for total hip replacements (THRs) are the posterior, transtrochanteric, direct lateral, and anterolateral approaches. Few publications describe the use of the anterior approach to do partial hip replacements or THRs [10, 11, 14]. In France, Judet and Judet [10] used Hueter's anterior approach since 1947 to implant neck replacements. They continued to use the anterior approach for THRs and spread the use of an approach derived from Hueter's approach, which removed the insertion of the tensor fasciae latae on the anterior iliac crest over 1–2 cm, sectioned the reflected tendon of the rectus femoris, and cut the piriformis muscle [11]. Since 1993 we have been using a minimally invasive anterior approach derived from this modified Hueter's approach. It allows for implantation of a total hip prosthesis with a 5- to 10-cm incision and no muscle or tendon section. It appeared to us that it was not necessary to perform any muscular or tendon section to obtain a good exposure. Postoperative rehabilitation is therefore simplified; the lack of muscular section allows quick indolence authorizing walking without

T. Siguier, MD (✉) • M. Siguier, MD • B. Brumpt, MD
Department of Orthopedic Surgery, Clinique Jouvenet,
6 Square Jouvenet, 75016 Paris, France
e-mail: thierry.siguier@9online.fr

D.G. Poitout, H. Judet (eds.), *Mini-Invasive Surgery of the Hip*,
DOI 10.1007/978-2-287-79931-0_1, © Springer France 2014

crutches. Furthermore a short skin incision (usually 6–8 cm) is sufficient in most cases, as long as during the procedure it is aided by the "hints and tricks" elaborated over a 17-year experience. This operative procedure, established by Marc Siguier and Bertrand Brumpt a long time before hip mini invasive surgery was in vogue, has systematically been used since June 1993. A large continuous series of 1,037 primary total hip replacements performed following this procedure between June 1993 and June 2000 has been reviewed retrospectively and published [23].

Anterior Approach and Hip Anatomy

The choice of an anterior approach for hip prosthetic surgery is anatomically logical. The anterior situation of the hip and the natural anteversion of the acetabulum and upper femur present them facing the surgeon for a patient in the supine position.

If seen from behind, the organization of muscular masses around the posterior part of the hip makes it in fact a deep articulation. This is because of the presence of the buttock muscles and the external rotators recovering the capsular plan. When considering the front part of the hip, the disposition of muscular masses allows for an intermuscular approach.

As reported by Lowell and Aufranc about [15] the Smith Petersen's approach, anterior approach "passes through an internervous line, the muscles medially being innervated by the femoral nerve and upper lumbar roots, those laterally being supplied by the superior gluteal nerve." The anterior approach is away from the sciatic nerve and the superior gluteal nerve.

Surgical Technique

The procedure we describe is reproducible and can be used for all patients with classic cases of osteoarthritis of the hip in which there is no previous surgical history. This technique has been used without navigation or an image intensifier.

Patient Positioning

The patient is always positioned in the dorsal decubitus position on a Judet's orthopedic table allowing traction, external and internal rotation, and lowering of the inferior limb foot to the ground during the procedure (Fig. 1.1a–c).

The sacrum rests on a scooped out pelvic support. This pelvic support stabilizes the pelvis and also allows for an efficient transmission of the orthopedic table's traction forces.

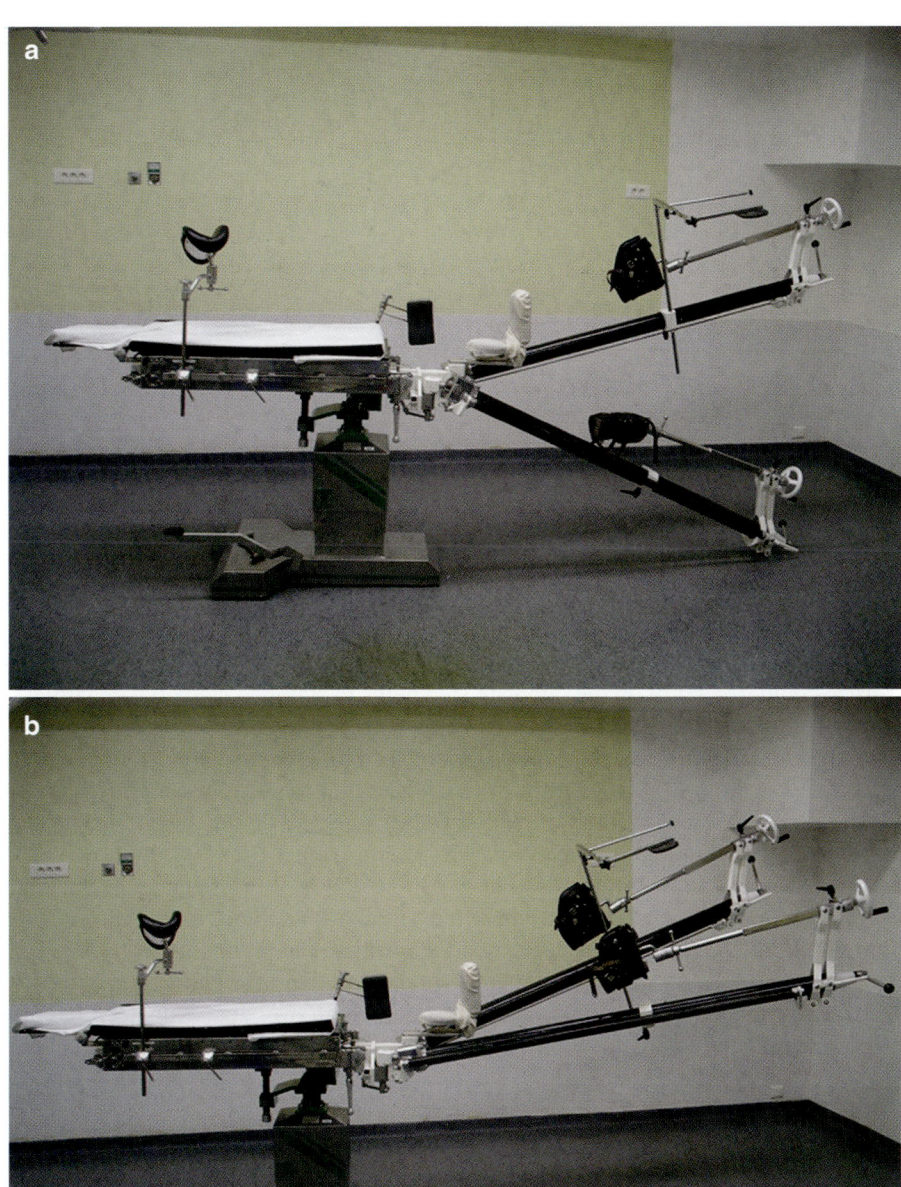

Fig. 1.1 (**a–c**) Judet's orthopedic table allowing a stable position of the pelvis and of the operated lower limb in the desired position

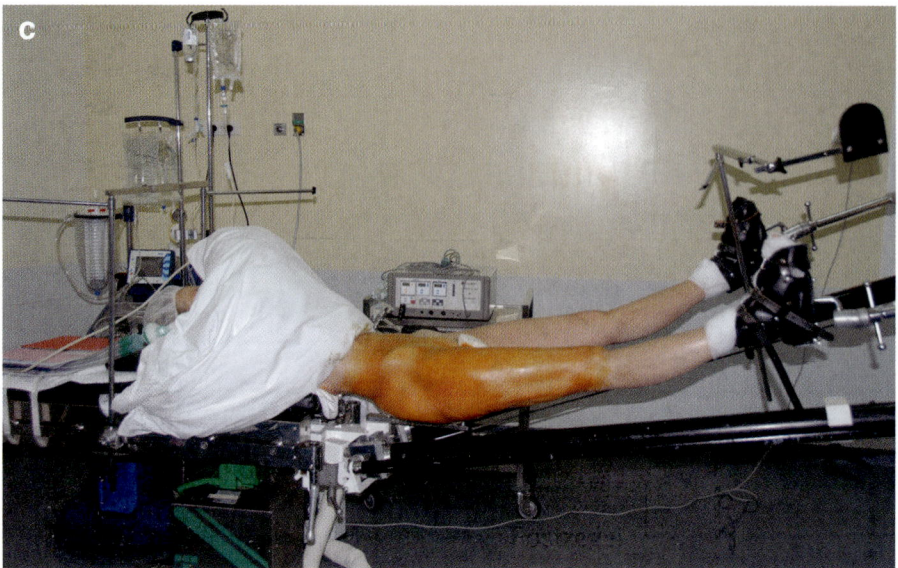

Fig. 1.1 (continued)

Iliac counterpressure on the opposite side helps to stabilize the pelvis regardless of the position of the limb being treated.

The opposite upper limb rests on a support, with the extended elbow. The operating side upper limb is positioned in front of the patient's chest, with a flexed forearm, in a way so as not to interfere with the surgeon's and first assistant's liberty of movements. Installation must be checked by the surgeon.

Two assistants help with surgery, but it can be done with just one assistant. The first assistant is positioned on the left of the surgeon for surgery on a right hip and on the right of the surgeon for surgery on a left hip. The second assistant is positioned opposite the surgeon. The operative field must expose the iliac crest in its anterior half and the anteroexternal surface of the thigh over approximately 20 cm.

For didactic purposes, the approach to the hip will be described in three planes.

Plane 1

The skin is incised parallel to an imaginary line joining the anterosuperior iliac spine to the head of the fibula. The incision is made approximately 2 cm behind this line (Fig. 1.2). The length of the skin incision ranges from 6 to 8 cm for a patient with normal body weight and can be increased in size if it does not provide sufficient comfort during surgery, particularly in obese or very muscular patients. It is rare to need an incision more than 10 cm long. With reference to the apex of the greater trochanter, which can be identified easily by palpation, the incision is made 2/3 above the apex and 1/3 below the apex (on the line described previously), that is, in

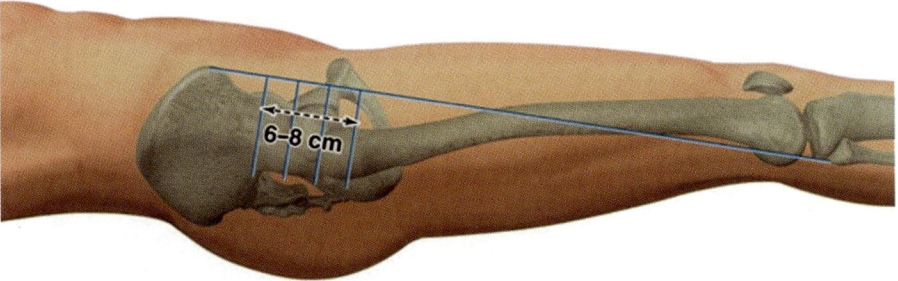

Fig. 1.2 The skin incision is positioned in reference to the apex of the greater trochanter and 2 cm behind an imaginary line joining the anterosuperior iliac spin to the head of the fibula

Fig. 1.3 The skin and fat tissue are incised to the superficial aponeurosis of the tensor fasciae latae

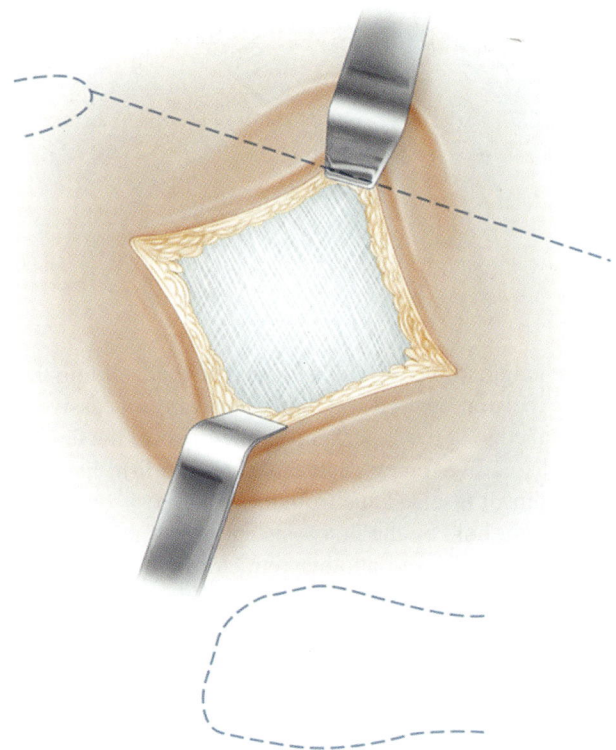

front of the greater trochanter (Fig. 1.3). After incising the subcutaneous fat and hemostasis, a buttonhole incision is made along the direction of the incision on the superficial aponeurosis of the tensor fasciae latae on the part which is most mobile on palpation. The correct location of the buttonhole incision is confirmed by the appearance of the muscle fibers, which are characterized because of their oblique path from above downward and from front to back (Fig. 1.4). The incision of the superficial aponeurosis of the tensor fasciae latae then is to be continued over the

Fig. 1.4 A buttonhole
incision is made on the
superficial aponeurosis of the
tensor fasciae latae along the
direction of the incision

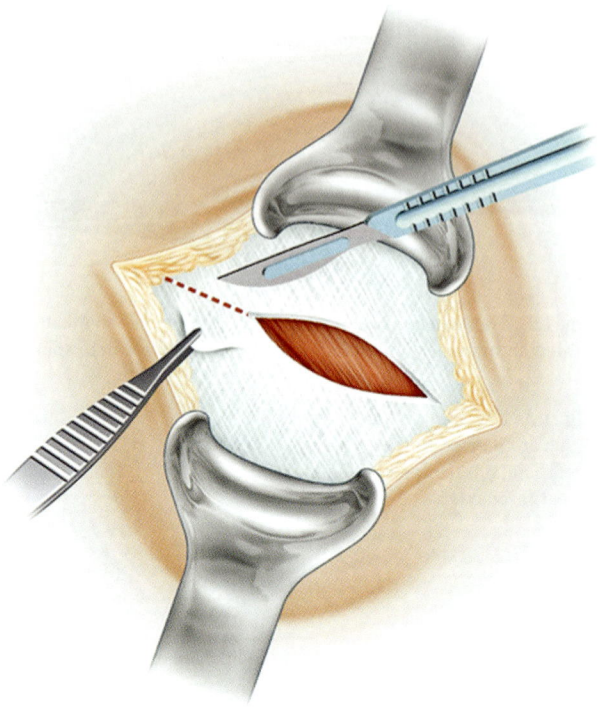

entire length of the skin incision and beyond, sliding the superior and inferior angles
of the incision upward and then downward successively using a small retractor. The
internal edge of the superficial aponeurosis of the tensor fasciae latae then is grasped
with dissecting forceps and raised with a firm hand to allow a rasp to release the
entire tensor fasciae latae from its aponeurosis over its anterointerior side (Fig. 1.5).
A retractor held by the first assistant then is used to displace the tensor fasciae latae
muscle laterally, and another retractor held by the second assistant is used to displace the sartorius muscle medially. Correctly balanced retraction then will allow
the second plane to be exposed perfectly.

Plane 2: Innominate Aponeurosis and Anterior Circumflex Vessels

This plane is located immediately on the deeper surface of the tensor fasciae latae
that is pulled aside by the first assistant. The innominate aponeurosis may be more
or less thick. The anterior circumflex vessels, which are visible beneath this aponeurosis, must be identified to tie them off or coagulate them. The presence of one or
two "sentinel" veins emerging at the superficial surface of the deep innominate
aponeurosis helps identify the bundle of circumflex vessels which vary in number,
volume, and location among patients. After these have been controlled (Fig. 1.6),

Fig. 1.5 The tensor fasciae latae muscle is released from its superficial aponeurosis after completely incising it

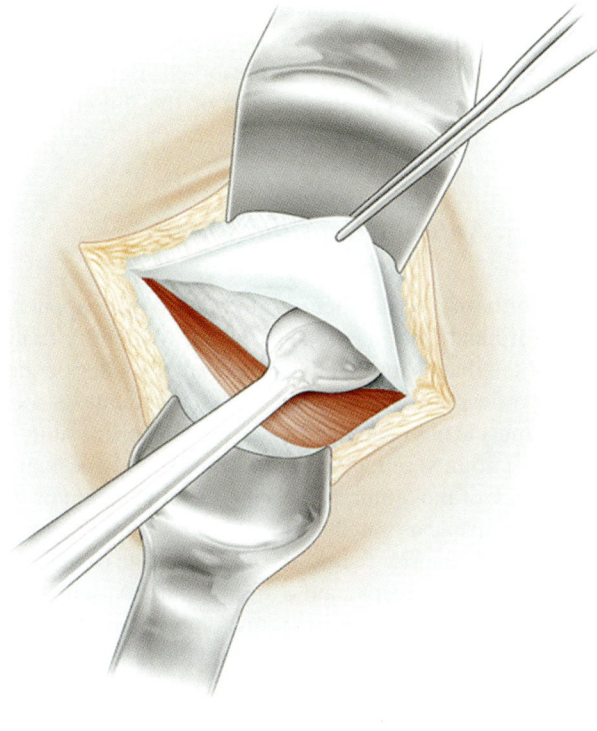

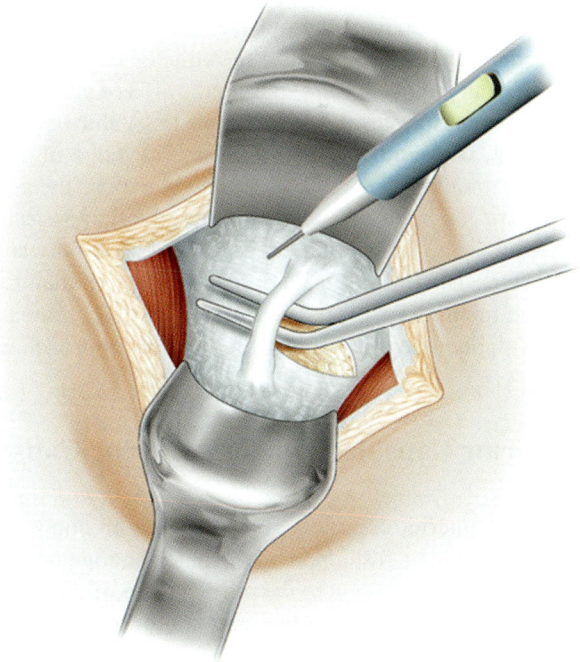

Fig. 1.6 The innominate aponeurosis and the anterior circumflex vessels are correctly exposed between the posterior retractor removing the tensor fasciae latae muscle and the anterior retractor removing the anterior rectus femoris muscle. The anterior circumflex vessels are ligated or coagulated

complete incision of the innominate aponeurosis may be done easily over the entire length of the incision. The incision begins upward at the level of the reflected tendon of the rectus femoris, which is preserved. Below, the aponeurosis becomes thinner and disappears. Complete incision of the innominate aponeurosis reveals a fatty space leading to the third plane.

Plane 3: Anterior Capsular Plane

The fatty tissue located beneath the innominate aponeurosis is incised from the top downward and from the outside inward to identify (without damaging) the aponeurosis of the iliacus muscle, which covers the anterior surface of the joint capsule to a greater or lesser extent depending on the patient. As soon as the external edge of the iliacus muscle has been identified, the thin perimysium which surrounds it is incised, and a first pointed retractor, held by the second assistant, is slid to the inferior surface of the neck of the femur, preserving the attachment of the iliacus muscle to the anterior joint capsule as much as possible. In its upper part, slightly beneath the reflected tendon of the anterior rectus, the external edge of the iliacus muscle is pulled upward with dissecting forceps, and a small white avascular space—the attachment of the direct tendon of the anterior rectus femoris onto the joint capsule—then can be dissected. A second pointed retractor, also held by the second assistant, is slid into this space. This then pulls aside the iliacus and rectus femoris muscles pressing on the anterior wall of the acetabulum. The retractor must be level with the anterior capsule and its insertion onto the anterior wall, beneath the two muscles described previously and not in the body of the muscle, to avoid the risk of damaging the femoral nerve with the pointed tip. Tilting the retractor exposes the inferior part of the anterior aspect of the joint capsule, sparing the area of attachment between the iliacus muscle and the anterior surface of the capsule. A third pointed retractor, held by the first assistant, will slide easily to the superior edge of the neck of the femur, between gluteus minimus and capsule, to clearly expose the anterior surface of the neck. The exposure can be improved even more: the first assistant who still has one free hand can pull aside the internal edge of the tensor, outward, with an American retractor (Fig. 1.7). The full surgical approach to the hip then is complete.

The methods of exposure and details that allow a total replacement to be done comfortably using this minimally invasive approach will be described.

Anterior Capsulectomy or Anterior Capsulotomy

Whether anterior capsulectomy is done with conventional or diathermal scalpel, a small lip must be fashioned on the anterior edge of the acetabulum. An internal flap which remains adherent to the deep surface of the iliacus muscle and protects it also must be made. This capsulectomy approximates 40 % of the surface of the whole capsule (Fig. 1.8).

Fig. 1.7 The exposed anterior capsule of the hip and the anterior capsulectomy are shown. The anterior retractor pulls aside the iliacus and rectus femoris muscles. The inferior retractor is slid to the inferior surface of the neck of the femur. The superior retractor is slid to the superior surface of the neck of the femur

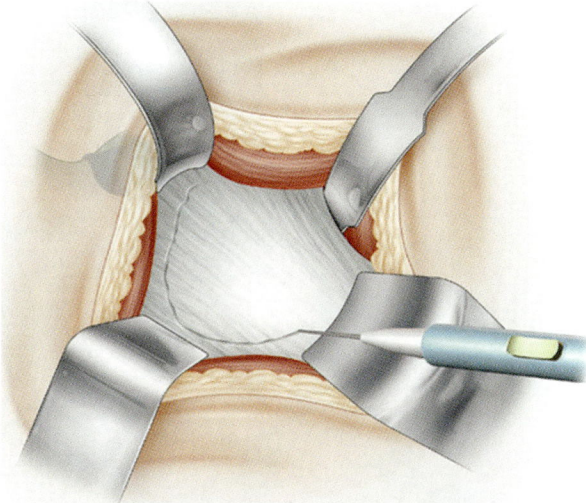

Fig. 1.8 The femoral head and neck are exposed after the partial anterior capsulectomy. The portion of excised anterior capsule is shown in the dissecting forceps

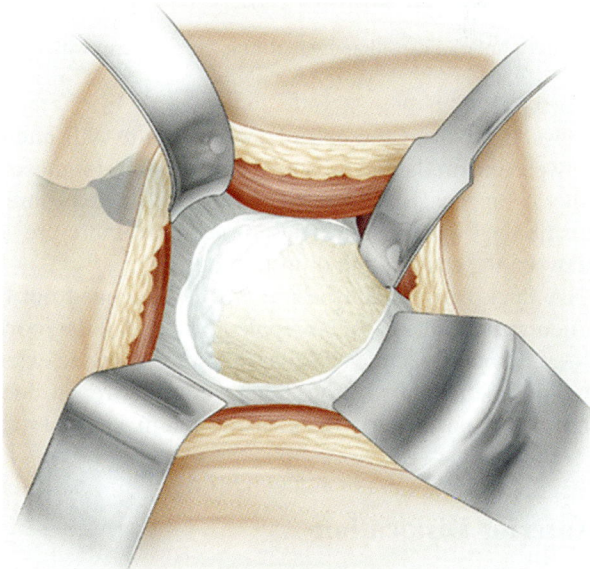

The anterior capsulectomy can be deliberately chosen by the surgeon. However, the capsulectomy must be performed in case of preoperative stiffness in extension, important stiffness, or in case of a planned shortening correction.

An anterior capsulotomy with a capsular repair at the end of the procedure can be done in all other cases. The capsulotomy will then be performed in a U-form with a superior acetabular hinge (Fig. 1.9). The exposure is made easier by the positioning of the curve retractor under the capsular flap, in contact with the anterior acetabulum's wall. This capsular flap protects the anterior muscles from the retractor.

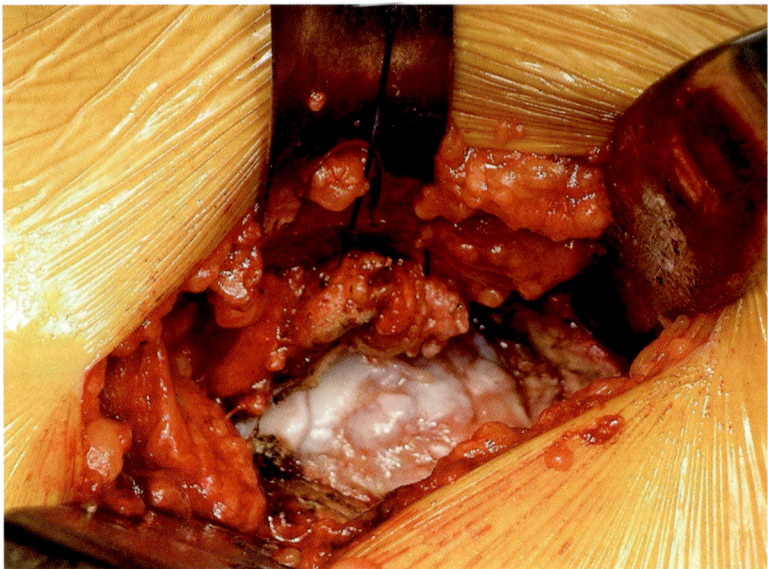

Fig. 1.9 Anterior capsulotomy performed in a U-form with a superior acetabular hinge

Capsular repair at the end of the procedure will allow to keep a protector tissue between the implanted prosthesis and the anterior muscles. However, even a reduced anterior approach allows a good acetabular exposure, hence an appropriate cup positioning without any edging, avoiding therefore a potential anterior conflict between the cup and the iliopsoas muscle.

A thick capsule can be preserved and tinned out by the resection of its deep articular side. The capsular repair, at the end of the procedure, is undertaken with an external rotation of the capsular flap sutured on the external capsulotomy zone, with the hip in external rotation. Such a capsular repair does not interfere with full hip movement, particularly in extension and in external rotation.

Anterior Dislocation

The femoral head is dislocated by external rotation after applying sufficient traction by means of the orthopedic table to insert a Lambotte spoon (Hospitalia, Fontenay les Briis, France) between the acetabulum and the femoral head (Fig. 1.10). After the Lambotte spoon has been inserted between the head and acetabulum, it is essential that the traction be released and that the limb is rotated with an assistant applying the rotation forces at the level of the knee, holding the knee below the surgical fields. The surgeon assists in dislocation by levering on the femoral head using the Lambotte spoon. A 90° external rotation must be obtained to estimate the anteversion of the femoral neck (Fig. 1.11). Femoral neck's cut is only performed after having checked that a 90° rotation is obtained by knee palpation. A condylar palpation

Fig. 1.10 A Lambotte spoon is inserted between the acetabulum and the femoral head before dislocation

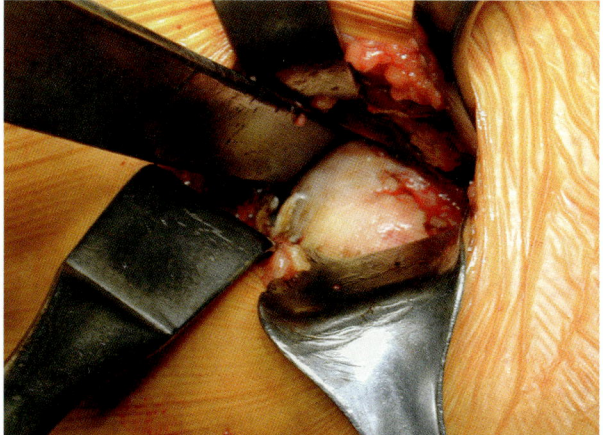

Fig. 1.11 The anterior dislocation is accomplished by external rotation and by levering onto the femoral head using the Lambotte spoon

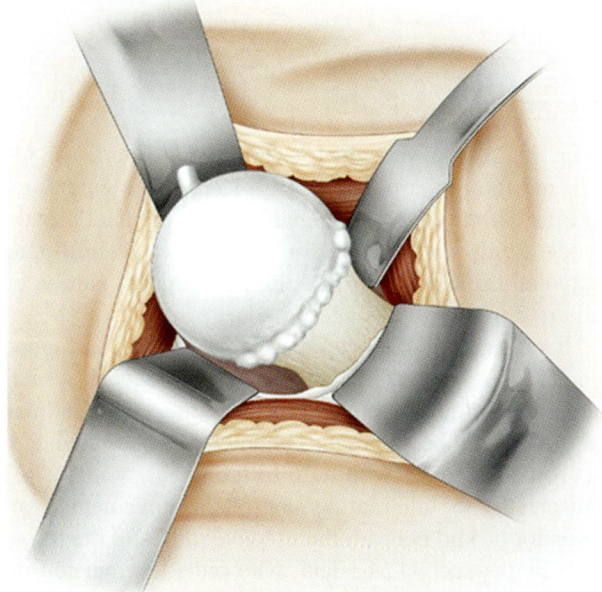

is more precise to assess rotation than a patellar palpation, especially where obese patients are concerned.

Femoral Neck's Cut

Identification of the height of the desired cut on the neck is achieved keeping the leg in 90° external rotation by comparing the length of the calculated resection from the preoperative template against the apex of the head using a caliper

Fig. 1.12 The level of
femoral neck section is
determined with a caliper

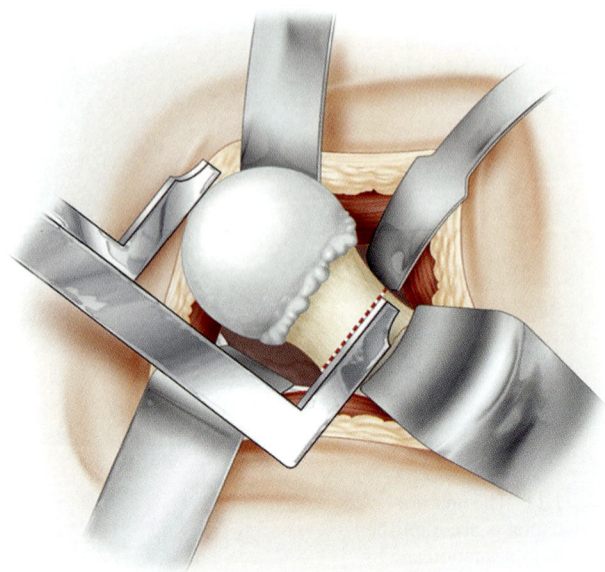

(Fig. 1.12). It is straight forward to reproduce the ideal length on a sterile caliper and to compare the length of resection calculated from preoperative radiographs with the apex of the head using the trial prosthesis. After the cut has been
made (with the caliper locked at the desired length), correct concordance
between the actual cut and the planned cut can be confirmed to be certain that
no error in length has been made.

Each surgeon can keep his planning and corresponding usual anatomical landmarks. The level of the planned femoral neck's section remains easy to assess
according to the surgeon habits as all the usual landmarks are easily accessible (tip
of the femoral head, great trochanter, lesser trochanter).

To cut the neck with an oscillating saw without risking damage to the skin or
muscles by the alternating saw blade movements, we recommend that a pointed
retractor be slid beneath the psoas tendon and the lesser trochanter. The retractor is
held by the second assistant, who pulls the incision downward. A second pointed
retractor is placed at the external side of the neck. The head of the femur disappears
partly beneath the upper portion of the incision, although the neck is remarkably
well exposed over its entire length.

Exposure of the lower part of the femoral neck before cutting may be improved
by an axial push of operated lower limb performed by the circulating nurse.

Soft tissues are protected by the two retractors (Fig. 1.13). The axis of the neck
of the femur then is exposed perfectly, helping to orientate the cut.

The femoral neck may also be cut in situ, without dislocation.

In this respect, the level of the cut is determined after visualization of the planned
cut level at the junction between the upper edge of the femoral neck and the medial

Fig. 1.13 The femoral neck
is cut with an oscillating saw

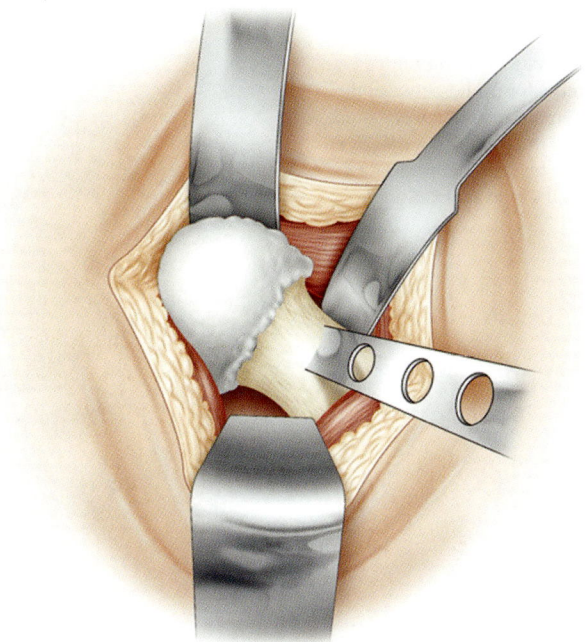

side of the greater trochanter. We prefer to cut the femoral neck after dislocation, which allows to perform a single neck cut according to plan. It also allows a precise choice of the anteversion of the cut.

Acetabulum Exposure

After releasing the rotation, the acetabulum generally is exposed perfectly by sliding a pointed retractor between the two horns of the acetabulum beneath the transverse ligament. This retractor pulls the iliopsoas muscle aside. A pointed retractor slid beneath the anterior wall of the acetabulum, as described previously pulls aside the iliacus muscle and the rectus femoris. The conservation of a capsular flap with a proximal acetabular hinge allows to insert an anterior retractor under that flap, directly on the anterior wall of the acetabulum. This capsular flap protects the anterior muscles from the retractor. These two retractors are held by the second assistant. A third pointed retractor is slid beneath the posterior wall and covers the stump of the neck and the tensor fasciae latae (Fig. 1.14). Sectioning of the posterior capsule is optional and is not required to expose the acetabulum. This is done only in case of severe preoperative stiffness or capsule hypertrophy.

The position of the acetabular component that we established is at a tilt between 40° and 45° in the frontal plane. Positioning in the frontal plane may be facilitated

Fig. 1.14 The acetabulum is
exposed with the anterior
retractor. The inferior
retractor is slid between the
two horns of the acetabulum,
and the posterior retractor is
slid beneath the posterior
wall of the acetabulum

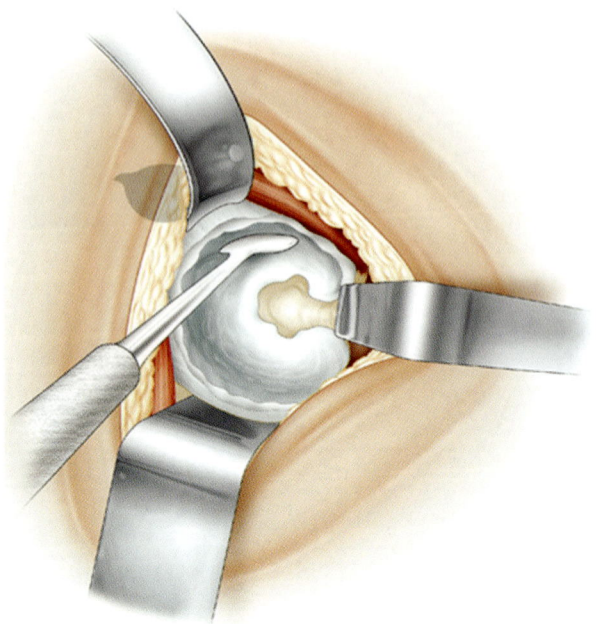

by palpating the two anterior iliac crests, which are easily accessible within the
operative field. We sought to produce slight anteversion of 10°–15° in the horizontal
plane. The desired position in the horizontal plane is easily assessed compared to
the horizontality of the floor.

Femoral Exposure

The lower limb again is locked at 90° or greater in external rotation. A retractor or
Lambotte spoon is slid level with the posterior side of the neck to provide better
exposure and is held by the second assistant. Application of traction allows the
greater trochanter to be released from the buttock. A pointed retractor then is slid to
the superior edge of the greater trochanter. This is held by the first assistant and
pulls the tensor fasciae latae aside and downward. The orthopedic table traction is
released gradually while the surgeon raises the trochanter upward, using his or her
fist, and applies pressure from below the buttock. The pressure is maintained while
the lower limb, locked at 90° external rotation, is lowered, foot to the ground
(Fig. 1.15).

The first assistant pulls aside the tensor fasciae latae with the pointed retractor,
and the surgeon releases the pressure when the superior tip of the femur is sufficiently
well exposed. This maneuver is necessary for exteriorization of the femur without
overstretching the tensor fasciae latae. Sectioning of the external rotators is avoided

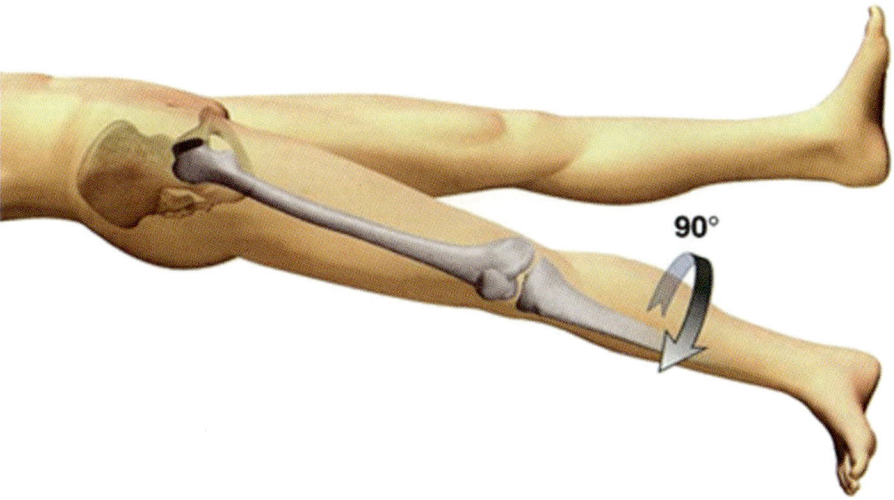

Fig. 1.15 The femoral canal is exposed by external rotation and lowering the lower limb, with the foot to the ground

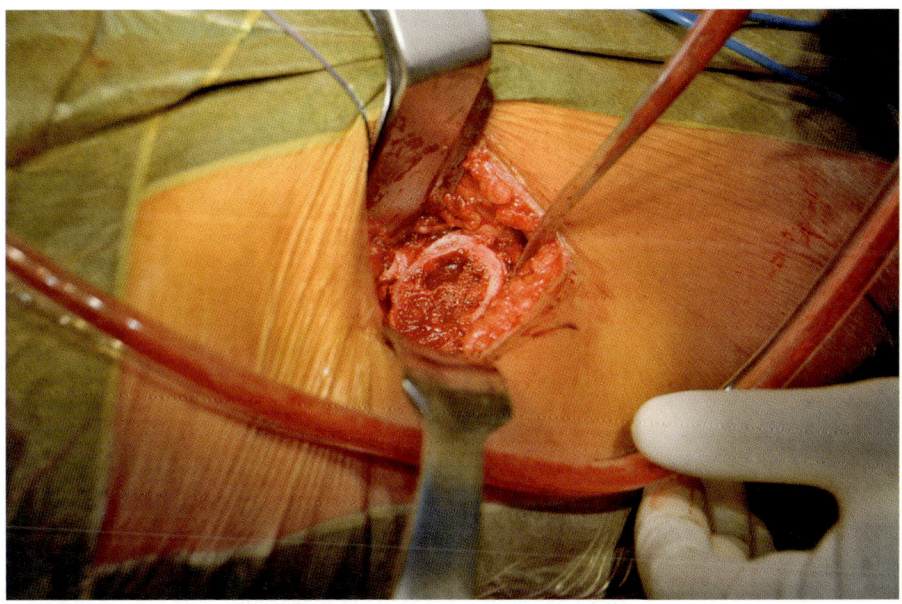

Fig. 1.16 Femoral exposure. Short external rotators are preserved totally

by the good femoral exposure that is obtained (Fig. 1.16). Additional superior capsulectomy sometimes is required to obtain correct exposure.

Superior capsulotomy is carried out from the superior edge of the greater trochanter to its posteroinferior angle. The femoral metaphysis is then well exposed,

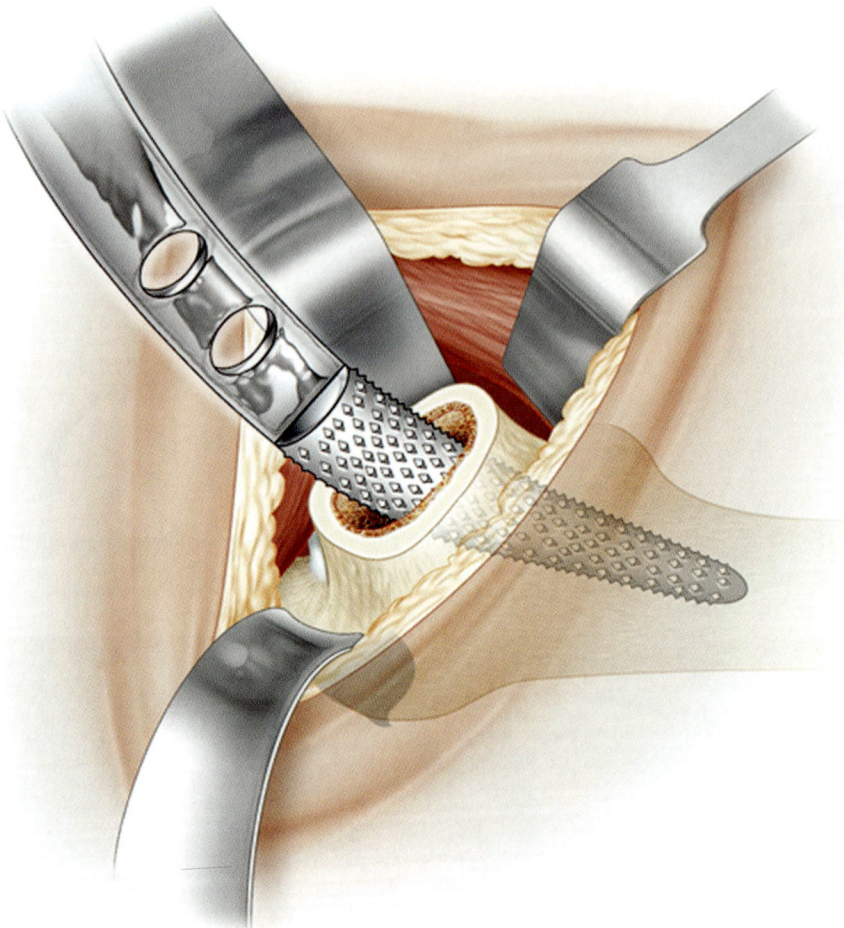

Fig. 1.17 The femoral canal is exposed, respecting the gluteus medius and the piriformis muscle

with an external rotation of 90° or greater, with a 20°–30° extension and with adduction. An axial push with the orthopedic table allows further exposure of the upper femur.

Gluteus medius and short external rotators are preserved totally, and the femur is well exposed to allow all of the maneuvers to implant the femoral prosthesis.

The femoral canal is prepared with reamers, the neck of which has an anterior angulation (Fig. 1.17). It is the only ancillary constraint of anterior approach.

A trial prosthesis is placed, and the femoral stem position is verified in relation to the apex of great trochanter (Fig. 1.18).

The femoral component is placed in 10°–15° anteversion.

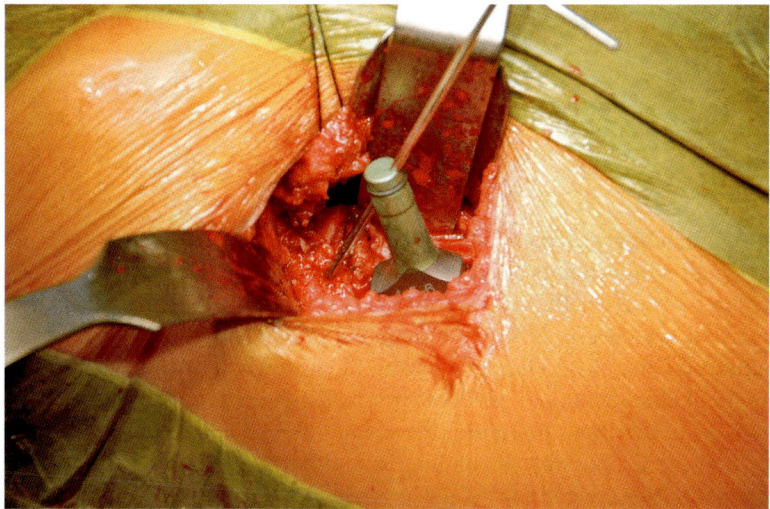

Fig. 1.18 Noncemented trial prosthesis in place, the femoral stem position is verified in relation to the apex of great trochanter

Fig. 1.19 Reduction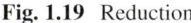

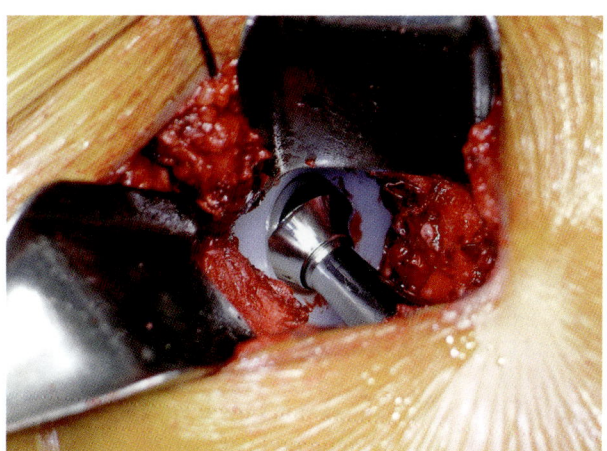

Reduction and Closure

Reduction is obtained by raising the leg traction then moving from 90° external rotation to the 0 position and relaxing traction for the femoral head to reenter the acetabulum (Fig. 1.19).

Closure is done in three planes: the superficial aponeurosis of the tensor, not going too far wide and inward to avoid damaging the cutaneous femoral nerve; the subcutaneous fatty tissue; and the skin then are sutured. An aspiration drain is kept in place until 2 or 3 days postoperatively.

Postoperative Care

Seated and standing positions are permitted the day after surgery. Active simple self-reeducation movements are done from the second day postoperatively. Patients are permitted to walk with full weightbearing on the first day. The decision to give up the use of crutches is left to the patient's judgement. Self-reeducation movements taught by the physiotherapist during the hospital stay are continued at home by the patient alone without a physiotherapist for the first 6 weeks postoperatively. Only patients living alone are referred to a rehabilitation home. In each case, patients returned home when possible depending on their family situation, in view of the fact that no functional reeducation was prescribed.

Retrospective Series: 1993–2000

We have previously reported a large retrospective series of total hip replacements performed by this anterior mini invasive approach to evaluate results, complications, and dislocation rate [23].

The minimally invasive anterior approach was used for the first time in 1993.

Between June 1993 and June 2000, 1,037 total primary arthroplasties were done in 926 patients using this technique. One hundred eleven bilateral procedures were done. Only hips that had not had any previous surgery before the THR were included in the study. Congenital posterior dislocated hips that required a more extensive approach were not included in the series nor were dysplastic hips, which had been operated on to produce an acetabular osteoplastic ridge or a superior femoral osteotomy.

Total hip replacements done for a fractured neck of the femur were excluded. Osteoarthritis was the main preoperative diagnosis (950 cases out of 1,037).

In each patient the implant used was Charnley's LFA MKII (Sanortho, Smith & Nephew, Orthez, France) with a 22.2-mm head. The femoral component was mono-block and made of stainless steel. The acetabular and femoral components were cemented in each patient. The cup used was a nonretaining, simple hemispheric cup without offset, made of ultrahigh molecular weight polyethylene (PE). The friction couple used in each patient was metal against PE.

All patients achieved full weightbearing on the surgically treated leg either the first or the second day postoperatively. Most patients were able to walk without crutches in their bedroom early postoperatively and on average discontinued using walking aids 8 days–3 weeks after the operation (among patients who previously had been walking without the support of two crutches). No cases of limp secondary to insufficiency of the gluteus medius were seen because the buttock muscles and greater trochanter were not affected by the surgical approach.

Two cases of postoperative femoralis paresis were observed. These resolved completely after 9 months and 1 year, respectively. One nondisplaced distal external malleolar fracture after manipulations on the orthopedic table occurred in an 87-year-old patient with severe osteoporosis. Postoperative care was not changed, and the patient was permitted to walk with complete weightbearing supported only by a simple elastic bandage. No revision surgery for hematoma was required, and no significant heterotopic ossification occurred. Septic complications occurred in five patients. Three cases of aseptic loosening were treated by a single-stage change of prosthesis. Ten of 1,037 hips dislocated (dislocation rate of 0.96 %). In eight of ten cases, the dislocation occurred in the first 2 months postoperatively, and in six cases it occurred during the first postoperative month. The dislocations were limited to one episode in seven patients and were recurrent in three patients.

Discussion

Since 1993 we have been systematically using the anterior, intermuscular planes minimally invasive approach to obtain early rehabilitation in patients needing total hip replacement.

The expected qualities of a surgical approach are preservation of the anatomy, quality of exposure, reproducibility, and possibilities of extension. All existing approaches for THR have their own advantages and disadvantages and anatomic structures that can be put at risk during exposure.

The minimally invasive anterior approach we describe is an anatomic route; it allows hip exposition and dislocation without any muscle or tendon sectioning. This approach is used without modification or extension to implant total noncemented prostheses.

The surgical approach is away from the sciatic nerve and the superior gluteal nerve. The femoral nerve is not seen in the approach, although it may be damaged by the anterior retractor, which must be positioned carefully under the iliopsoas muscle.

The lateral femoral cutaneous nerve is not put at risk with skin incision due to the external displacement of the approach which is made in the tensor fasciae latae aponeurosis. The lateral femoral cutaneous nerve's preservation is facilitated by the incision's direction and its external position with regard to the anterosuperior iliac spin. Great care must be taken during closure, in order not to damage the lateral femoral cutaneous nerve, by not going too far into the internal lip of the aponeurosis of tensor fasciae latae muscle.

Obesity is not a contraindication for the minimally invasive anterior approach, which does not require a preoperative decision regarding its use. In case of exposure difficulties, the length of the skin incision can be increased to facilitate the exposure.

The hip approach continues with the same technique using only intermuscular planes, preserving muscles and tendons. The excess of fatty tissue does not impede muscular preservation. On the contrary, important muscular masses on men with large body frames can indicate sectioning of the piriformis muscle is needed for correct upper-femoral exposure. It very rarely happens, the posterior capsulotomy is normally sufficient to obtain a good femoral exposure.

Immediate return to walking with complete weightbearing is facilitated by preserving the trochanter and all the abductor muscles. Self-rehabilitation is sufficient and is based on simple exercises, including active abduction exercises without the need for a physiotherapist or a stay in a rehabilitation center.

Orthopedic Table

The quality of exposure is excellent for the acetabular cavity, which is facing the surgeon because of its anatomic anteversion, with the retractors allowing for complete removal of the muscle masses from the field of vision. A proper acetabular cup position with the desired anteversion and abduction angle is facilitated by having patients lie in the supine position. The pelvis is stable because it is fixed firmly by the pelvic support and by iliac counterpressure. This stability of the pelvis, which is not changed by the exposure and retraction maneuvers, allows reliable positioning of the acetabular component. The two femoral crests are very easy to access on palpation, which may facilitate orientation of the acetabular component in the frontal plane. Anteversion of the acetabular cup is evaluated easily because of excellent exposure of the acetabulum and with reference to the ground.

The neck of the femur is visible directly by the surgeon, allowing adjustment of anteversion of the femoral component. The adjustment is controlled by assessing rotation of the knee at 90° external rotation. All these maneuvers are facilitated by the use of a Judet's orthopedic table.

The hip can be mobilized in all directions, flexion-extension, abduction-adduction, and rotations. Femoral exposure in particular is facilitated by the foot to the ground position, with extension of the hip.

The limb in question is maintained and supported by the orthopedic table, thus freeing the surgeon's assistants from this task.

Total hip replacement using the Hueter's or Watson Jones' approach also can be done without an orthopedic table [14].

The patient is then installed in decubitus dorsal or lateral on an ordinary operating table. However, certain situations can make the exposure of the upper femur more difficult, for example, with certain highly muscled patients or certain anatomic configurations of the femoral neck as coxa vara or retrorsa or reversed iliac wing. In these situations, the interest of using an orthopedic table to ease the femoral exposure becomes evident compared to an anterior approach performed on an ordinary table.

Possibilities of Extension

Subsequent surgical revision using the same approach with widening is possible when required. Proximal widening is performed according to Smith Petersen's approach. Distal widening to the femoral diaphysis is performed according to Zahradnicek's approach. Another possibility is to perform a second femoral diaphysis direct approach without having to extend the existing anterior approach.

Hip Stability

Postoperative dislocation after THR occurs at an incidence of between 2 % and approximately 10 % according to Kelley [12]. The occurrence of dislocation after THA is a worrisome and potentially serious problem. According to Hedlund et al. [8], after an initial dislocation of a Charnley's prosthesis with a 22.2-mm head, 35 % of hips do not have a recurrence of dislocation. Results of the treatment for recurrent dislocations after THA are disappointing [5, 7–9, 17]. The choice of an approach that does not increase the risk of dislocation therefore is important. Numerous authors agree on the correlation between positioning of prosthetic components and the presence of instability [3, 6, 13, 16, 19]. Our 0.96 % dislocation rate for 1,037 Charnley's monoblock prosthesis, with a 22.2-mm femoral head and with a standard nonretaining cup, is an indirect indicator of the quality of exposure offered by this minimal approach, which allows good control of the positioning of the prosthetic components. Despite the reduced size of the approach, minimally anterior approach for THR does not increase dislocation rate. We deduct that this minimally invasive approach allows for correct positioning of the two prosthetic components. The low dislocation rate is an indirect indicator of this. Preserving the muscular potential contributes also probably to the dynamic stabilization of the hip.

   Numerous authors have reported technical modifications designed to repair the muscle and tendon or bone structures in the case of trochanterotomy, damaged during the surgical approach, including repairs to the external rotators for the posterior approach, [1, 18, 20] or either modified or limited trochanterotomy [2, 4] with the same aim.

Conclusion

This minimally invasive anterior approach using intermuscular planes allows a surgical approach to the hip and implantation of a total hip prosthesis with no muscle, tendon, or trochanteric section, even partially. This is not offered by any other surgical approach. Preserving the abductors and gluteal muscles with an approach that is distant to them avoids the risk of limp attributable to insufficiency of the gluteus medius. The anatomy aspect is more important for us than the unquestionable cosmetic advantage obtained by the reduced size of the incision.

We also used this limited approach to implant a single femoral or total arthroplasty for fractured neck of femur using identical methodology with preservation of the anterior capsule, the anterior capsulotomy being sutured at the end of the procedure. This approach also has been used to implant partially resurfaced implants for osteonecrosis of the femoral head [21, 22]. Systematic use of this mini invasive anterior approach for THR is not jeopardized by a higher complication rate than the habitual anterior approach [23].

The low incidence of dislocation is an indirect indication of the fact that the acetabular and femoral implants have been positioned according to the surgeon's wishes, as well as a possible indication of the importance of preserving the soft tissues. The minimally invasive anterior approach for THR is a safe and reproducible technique providing low morbidity and fast postoperative recovery.

References

1. Chiu FY, Chen CM, Chung TY, Lo WH, Chen TH (2000) The effect of posterior capsulorrhaphy in primary total hip arthroplasty. J Arthroplasty 15:194–199
2. Courpied JP, Desportes G, Postel M (1991) Une nouvelle trochantérotomie pour l'abord postéro-externe de la hanche. Rev Chir Orthop 77:506–512
3. Coventry MB, Beckenbaugh RD, Nolan RD, Ilstrup DM (1974) 2012 total hip arthroplasties: a study of postoperative course and early complications. J Bone Joint Surg 56A:273–284
4. Dall D (1986) Exposure of the hip by anterior osteotomy of the greater trochanter: a modified anterolateral approach. J Bone Joint Surg 68B:382–386
5. Daly PJ, Morrey BF (1992) Operative correction of an unstable total hip arthroplasty. J Bone Joint Surg 74A:1334–1343
6. Fackler CD, Poss R (1980) Dislocation in total hip arthroplasties. Clin Orthop 151:169–178
7. Goetz DD, Capello WN, Callaghan JJ, Brown TD, Johnston RC (1998) Salvage of a recurrently dislocating total hip prosthesis with use a constrained acetabular component. J Bone Joint Surg 80A:502–509
8. Hedlundh U, Sanzén L, Fredin H (1997) The prognosis and treatment of dislocated total hip arthroplasties with a 22mm head. J Bone Joint Surg 79B:374–378
9. Hedlundh U, Hybbinette CH, Fredin H (1995) Influence of surgical approach on dislocations after Charnley hip arthroplasty. J Arthroplasty 10:609–614
10. Judet J, Judet R (1950) The use of an artificial femoral head for arthroplasty of the hip joint. J Bone Joint Surg 32B:166–173
11. Judet J, Judet H (1985) Voie d'abord antérieure dans l'arthroplastie totale de hanche. Presse Med 14:1031–1033
12. Kelley SS, Lachiewicz PF, Hickman JM, Paterno SM (1998) Relationship of femoral head and acetabular size to the prevalence of dislocation. Clin Orthop 355:163–171
13. Lewinnek GE, Lewis JL, Tarr R, Compere CL, Zimmerman JR (1978) Dislocations after total hip arthroplasties. J Bone Joint Surg 60A:217–220
14. Light TR, Keggi KJ (1980) Anterior approach to hip arthroplasty. Clin Orthop 152:255–260
15. Lowell JD, Aufranc OE (1968) The anterior approach to the hip joint. Clin Orthop 61:193–198
16. Morrey BF (1997) Difficult complications after hip joint replacement: dislocation. Clin Orthop 344:179–187
17. Parvizi J, Morrey BF (2000) Bipolar hip arthroplasty as a salvage treatment for instability of the hip. J Bone Joint Surg 82A:1132–1139

18. Pellici PM, Bostrom M, Poss R (1998) Posterior approach to total hip replacement using enhanced posterior soft tissue repair. Clin Orthop 355:224–228
19. Ritter MA (1976) Dislocation and subluxation of the total hip replacement. Clin Orthop 121:92–94
20. Robinson RP, Robinson HJ Jr, Salvati EA (1980) Comparison of the transtrochanteric and posterior approaches for total hip replacement. Clin Orthop 147:143–147
21. Siguier M, Judet T, Siguier T et al (1999) Preliminary results of partial surface replacement of the femoral head in osteonecrosis. J Arthroplasty 14:45–51
22. Siguier T, Siguier M, Judet T, Charnley G, Brumpt B (2001) Partial resurfacing arthroplasty of the femoral head in avascular necrosis: methods, indications, and results. Clin Orthop 386:85–92
23. Siguier T, Siguier M, Brumpt B (2004) Mini incision anterior approach does not increase dislocation rate: a study of 1037 total hip replacements. Clin Orthop 426:164–173

Chapter 2
Mini-Invasive Approach and Navigation in Total Prosthesis of the Hip

Henri Judet

Abstract The anterior approach to the hip, initially described by Hueter, has been modified and used by Jean and Robert Judet since 1947 for fixing an acrylic prosthesis rendering this approach completely mini-invasive by avoiding any muscular disinsertion or sectioning of tendons [1]. When we learnt about the possibilities of using the navigation technique for a hip prosthesis using the OrthoPilot system, we decided to combine these two innovations so as to induce a minimum of aggression and a maximum of security while fixing a hip prosthesis.

A study carried out on the positioning of the acetabulum, with or without navigation, as well as a comparison between two navigation systems attempts to validate the accuracy of the procedure.

Keywords Total hip replacement • Anterior approach • Mini-invasive surgery • Navigation technique

Introduction

We believe that combination of two innovative concepts, the mini-invasive approach and the navigation technique, would revolutionise the surgery of hip prosthesis.

We are quite familiar with the mini-invasive anterior approach [2] since this technique has been used in our practice since 1993. Being a modification of the technique used by Hueter, its principle is based on the nondetachment and non-sectioning of any muscles or tendons [3]. The navigation technique was adopted 6 years ago by the use of the OrthoPilot system developed by the B. Braun–Aesculap laboratory [4] and by the Amplivision system of the amplitude laboratory since 3 years.

H. Judet
Department of Orthopaedic, Clinique Jouvenet,
6 Square Jouvenet, 75016 Paris, France
e-mail: henri.judet@orange.fr

D.G. Poitout, H. Judet (eds.), *Mini-Invasive Surgery of the Hip*,
DOI 10.1007/978-2-287-79931-0_2, © Springer France 2014

In this work, we will describe the technique of the approach and of the navigation. We mention the results of a comparative study with and without navigation for positioning the acetabular part, and we attempt to validate the frame of reference by comparing the two systems of navigation used.

Surgical Technique

Positioning of the Patient

- The patient is placed in a dorsal decubitus on the Judet's orthopaedic table.
- A liquid-level gauge enables one to ensure that both limbs are in a horizontal position.
- Electrocardiogram electrode aids are fixed on the iliac spine opposite the side to be operated and on the pubis to serve as reference points under the fields during the acquisition of the pelvis plane.
- Two helpers are necessary, one on the side of the operator and the other in front of him.
- The computer equipped with its camera is placed on the opposite side facing the operator.

Preparation for Navigation

- A pin is fixed vertically on the iliac crest at a distance of three fingers behind the anterosuperior iliac spine so as not to hinder future manoeuvres during the introduction of the prosthesis in the femoral diaphysis.
- A second pin is placed in the femoral shaft with a bicortical grip and oriented from inside towards the outside on the internal side of the thigh at its inferior third through the medial great in a manner that the diode that it will bear faces the camera in a 90° external rotation.
- Both pins will bear passive diodes.
- Then the plane of the pelvis (Lewineck's plane) is acquired from the anterosuperior iliac spine and the pubis.

Mini-Invasive Anterior Approach

- The cutaneous incision straddles the hip's flexion fold in the direction of the anterosuperior iliac spine head of the fibula. It usually runs along a distance of

6–8 cm but may be stretched for obese subjects or for those having a stout muscle structure.

- Having pushed back the subcutaneous fat, incision of the superficial aponeurosis of the fascia lata's tensor is carried out. Following this and between the internal side of this aponeurosis and the muscle body, a natural fatty space is found leading directly to the anterior side of the capsule without causing any damage to tendons or to muscles. The internal edge of the aponeurosis reclining backwards protects the femoral cutaneous nerve that is the main obstacle to this approach.
- Only the anterior circumflex pedicle that crosses the incision at its lower part is to be coagulated.
- Then, an anterior flap of the articular capsule is excised to uncover the head and neck of the femur.
- With the help of the orthopaedic table, a Lambotte's spoon is introduced under traction, and after releasing the traction, the head of the femur is dislocated by rotating the lower limb over 90°. The helper who manipulates the orthopaedic table must always carry out the external rotation by guiding the limb over the knee so as to avoid any distortion of this joint.
- The neck may then be sectioned to the length calculated at the operation planning stage using an oscillating saw, and this length is attained with the help of a calliper.

Navigated Fixation of the Acetabulum

- The inferior limb must be left free to rotate. A jaw retractor having a precise curvature is placed between the two horns of the acetabulum, a second jaw retractor is positioned on the posterior edge and a third flat retractor brings the right anterior forward without hindering the crural nerve.
- Once the acetabular cavity is well exposed, the background level is obtained for navigation through a few points after removing its osteophytes, if present.
- Then, the centre of the acetabulum is situated using a test acetabulum of size inferior to that of the final acetabulum.
- Boring is then carried out progressively using reamers of increasing sizes until the one chosen at planning stage is reached. During reaming, the computer permanently indicates the angle and anteversion orientation in comparison to the previously defined plane of the pelvis. The computer also indicates the depth of boring in relation to the background.
- The test acetabula followed by the final acetabulum are impacted by always controlling the orientation chosen by the operator.
- The insert is fixed when the impacted acetabulum is steady. A test sphere connected to a sensor is used with rotating movements to provide the computer with the new centre of the acetabulum.
- The positioning of the femoral part will be obtained from the orientation and the new centre of the acetabulum.

Navigated Fixation of the Femoral Prosthesis

- The entrance of the femoral canal is exposed using an orthopaedic table and by lowering the inferior limb to ground level through hyperextension, adduction and 90° external rotation. All traction should be released to avoid any threat to the crural or sciatic nerves.
- A proper exposure of the entrance of the canal might require the resection of the superior capsule between the section of the cervix and the greater trochanter, without, in any case, sectioning the trochanterian pelvis that is quite often visible. A double jaw retractor is placed along the external surface of the greater trochanter for better exposure of the entrance of the femoral canal. A maximum of adduction is to be exerted to avoid conflict between the handle of the rasp and the pin of the iliac crest.
- The computer tracks the orientation of the femoral rasp according to the orientation of the acetabulum placed earlier. Due to its freedom in the canal, the first rasp allows regulation of the anteversion such that the cone of optimal mobility, indicated by the computer, is observed from the inside, without any risk of luxation or conflict. The subsequent rasps would then follow the same tract and would each time be controlled by the software.
- Once the last rasp is fixed, a test sphere is placed and reduction is executed by using the orthopaedic table.
- The software then allows control over the length and the offset. The length of the cervix can be modified if the result is not confirmed (three lengths with 3.5 mm gaps between each) or the offset (a six lateralised head) till reaching the best compromise for re-establishing the functional anatomy of the patient's hip as best possible.
- The final femoral prosthesis is then fixed while the computer verifies that the thrusting of the prosthesis is identical to that of the rasp.
- Once the head has been set in place and the reduction performed, a new final control of the length and of the offset is possible.

Closure of the Mini-Invasive Approach

- Closure is easy. It is only necessary to suture both edges of the superficial aponeurosis of the tensor of the fascia lata, carryout a levelling of the subcutaneous fat and suture the skin, which generally requires 7–8 points, or perform an intradermal continuous suture.
- Postoperative drainage is maintained for 48 h and the spica for 12 h following the intervention.

Postoperative Sequels

- As from the next day, the patient may move in a wheelchair and may get recourse to aided walking on the second or third day depending on the patient's general state.
- Hospitalisation lasts 6–8 days.
- A treatment with an anticoagulant is extended to 6 weeks.

Results

The mini-invasive approach as practised by us allows simple and quick sequels:

- Resumption of rest as from the second or third day
- Drainage: 2 days
- Bleeding from 6 to 800 cc
- Postoperative pain for the first 48 h, EVA 4/10
- Average hospitalisation of 8 days.

Does Navigation Improve the Positioning of the Acetabular Part?

Thirty-eight navigated insertions were compared to 40 conventional insertions. When measuring the anteversion and the gradient, the difference between both techniques is not significant, but the navigated group displays a less important standard deviation, thus testifying a better reproducibility of the positioning.

Is the Reference Plane Used and Transmitted by the Computer Reliable?

Two navigation systems were compared in an attempt to answer this fundamental question: on one hand, the OrthoPilot navigation system using the Lewineck's plane [5] and, on the other hand, the Amplivision navigation system using the plane of the femur in a neutral upright position. Both systems are designed to evaluate conflict zones according to the relative orientation of the two parts. Sixty-nine cases using the Lewineck's plane were compared to 31 cases using the femur plane. The sum of the shaft plus acetabulum anteversions that allows remaining in the safety zone is identical, 32° and 31°.

If one of the components has an excessive orientation in anteversion at the start, the second component rectifies in an identical way:

- If the anteversion of the acetabulum in the Lewineck's plane is above 25°, the shaft is oriented under 10°.
- If the anteversion of the shaft in the femur plane is above 20°, the acetabulum is oriented under 15°.

The choice of the pelvic or femoral frame of reference does not seem to influence the assessment of the mobility cone by navigation and thus the risk of conflict between the different prosthetic parts.

Discussion

Even if it is granted that experienced surgeons usually fix their prosthesis correctly, there is a certain margin of error capable of seriously influencing the results in the long run [6]. This study, like others, seems to demonstrate a better reproducibility of the positioning by using navigation [7].

But the experiments are still short and certain parameters were not taken into account, like the position of the pelvis compared to the lumbar spine in different positions of everyday life (walking, sitting, stepping, etc.).

Moreover, the use of a scanner to measure the postoperative position of the acetabulum has certain limits, considering the difference in planes between the surgical position and the position during the scan.

Further studies need thus to be carried out to validate the advantage of using navigation when fixing a hip prosthesis.

Conclusion

The simultaneous use of a mini-invasive anterior approach and navigation seems to provide the best surgical approach for a total hip prosthesis.

The mini-invasive approach provides better immediate sequels of functional recovery and reduces pain and bleeding.

Navigation seems to provide a better reproducibility in fixing implants and in giving security to the mobility cone against luxations and conflicts. The time for a proper hindsight remains very short and the equipment and reference frame works too perfectible for a proper validation of the benefits of navigation.

References

1. Judet J, Judet R (1950) The use of an artificial femoral head for arthroplasty of the hip joint. J Bone Joint Surg Br 32B(2):166–173
2. Judet J, Judet H (1985) Voie d'abord anterieure dans l'arthroplastie totale de hanche. Presse Med 14:1031–1033
3. Siguier T, Siguier M, Brumpt B (2004) Mini-incision anterior approach does not increase dislocation rate: a study of 1037 total hip replacements. Clin Orthop Relat Res 426:164–173
4. Judet H (2007) Five years' of experience in hip navigation using a mini-invasive anterior approach. Orthopaedics 30(10 Suppl):S141–S143
5. Lewineck GE, Lewis JL, Tarr R et al (1978) Dislocation after total hip replacement arthroplasties. J Bone Joint Surg Am 60:217–220
6. Kennedy JG, Roger WB, Soffe KE et al (1998) Effect of acetabular component orientation on recurrent dislocation, pelvic osteolysis, polyethylene wear and component migration. J Arthroplasty 13(5):530–534
7. Kalteis T, Handel M, Herold T et al (2005) Greater accuracy in positioning of the acetabular cup by using an image free navigation system. Int Orthop 29(5):272–276

Chapter 3
Anterior Hueter-Type Approach in Lateral Decubitus on a Conventional Table

Gilles Wepierre

Abstract The anterior Hueter approach, adapted for hip arthroplasty by J. and R. Judet, has become mini-invasive since the works of M. Siguier, who devised a technique to avoid any tendon or muscle section. It is usually performed in dorsal decubitus on an orthopaedic table.

Our approach does not require the use of an orthopaedic table (OT); the patient is positioned in lateral decubitus on a conventional table with the posterior distal half removed. Specific ancillary instrumentation is essential for each acetabular and femoral phase for precise positioning of the implants and to minimise soft tissue damage.

This enables an apical arthrotomy with preservation of the anterior capsular plane.

Keywords Total hip replacement • Mini-invasive surgery • Anterior approach • Lateral decubitus

Introduction

After extensive experience with posterior and then transgluteal approaches, we logically arrived at the Roettinger approach, which we have been practicing for over 2 years. The desire to reduce mechanical damage to the gluteus medius from the reamers and to preserve innervation of the TFL at the medial angle of the incision leads us to an approach from the front of the body of the TFL via the interneural space described by Hueter. The benefit of lateral decubitus for the acetabulum and an arthrotomy that spares the anterior capsular plane could thus be combined with the muscle and nerve-sparing benefits of the Hueter approach (Fig. 3.1). A specific

G. Wepierre
Department of Orthopedics,
Clinique La Ligne Bleue Epinal, Epinal, France
e-mail: gwepierre@wanadoo.fr

D.G. Poitout, H. Judet (eds.), *Mini-Invasive Surgery of the Hip*,
DOI 10.1007/978-2-287-79931-0_3, © Springer France 2014

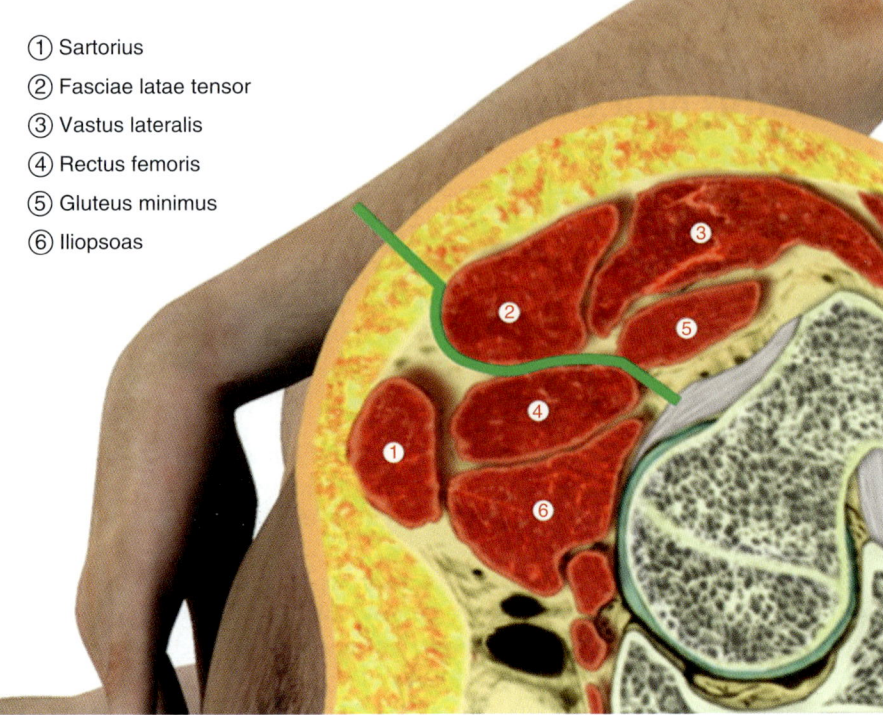

1. Sartorius
2. Fasciae latae tensor
3. Vastus lateralis
4. Rectus femoris
5. Gluteus minimus
6. Iliopsoas

Fig. 3.1 Route of the Hueter approach

femoral instrument has been developed to bypass the muscle mass of the TFL whilst limiting proximal femoral stress.

In this chapter, we present the surgical technique and our results and discuss the advantages and disadvantages of the concept.

Surgical Technique

General anaesthesia is preferable in athletic patients to achieve optimal myorelaxation.

The level of neuromuscular blockade following curarisation is checked prior to the femoral phase, and there is close collaboration with the anaesthetists.

Installation

The patient is placed in lateral decubitus on a conventional operating table with the posterior distal section removed.

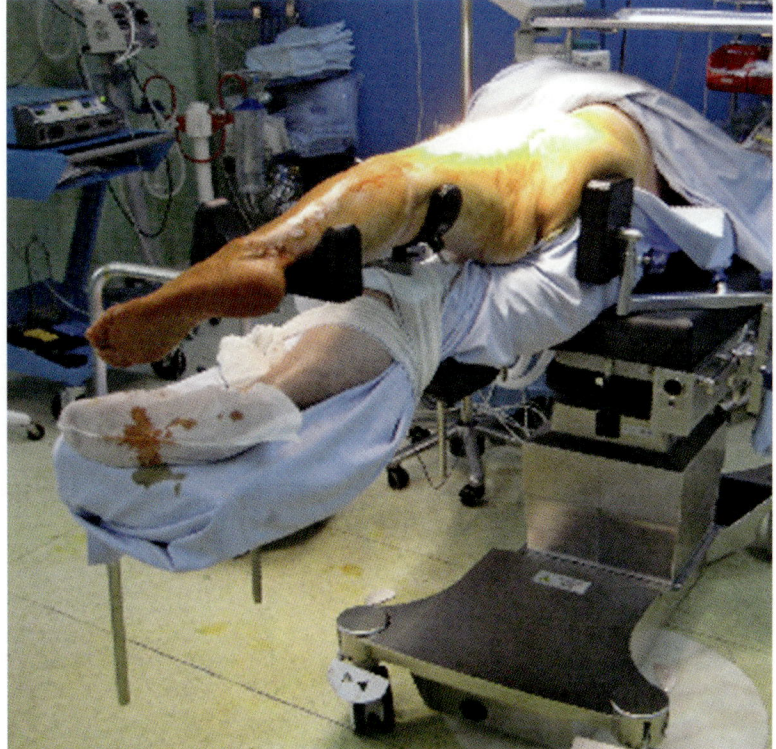

Fig. 3.2 Patient installation in lateral decubitus on a conventional table

The pelvis is stabilised for an anterior approach with support to the sacrum and pubis; the hip is flexed at 15°.

The lower extremity rests on two supports, one supracondylar and the other under the distal fourth of the leg. The posterior space enables luxation of the limb with complete freedom of movement using its weight alone in external rotation, extension, and adduction (Fig. 3.2).

A sterile bag is placed behind during the femoral phase, protecting the leg held vertically.

Incision

The oblique incision, 8–10 cm in length, is made over the neck of the femur along a line running from the anterior-superior iliac spine two fingerbreadths from the summit of the greater trochanter (Fig. 3.3).

Fig. 3.3 Oblique incision
from the anterior-superior
iliac spine to summit of the
greater trochanter

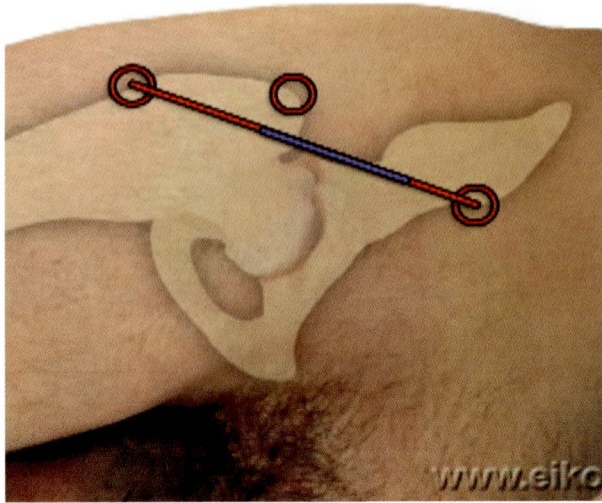

Fig. 3.4 Incision of the
aponeurosis of the tensor
fasciae lata

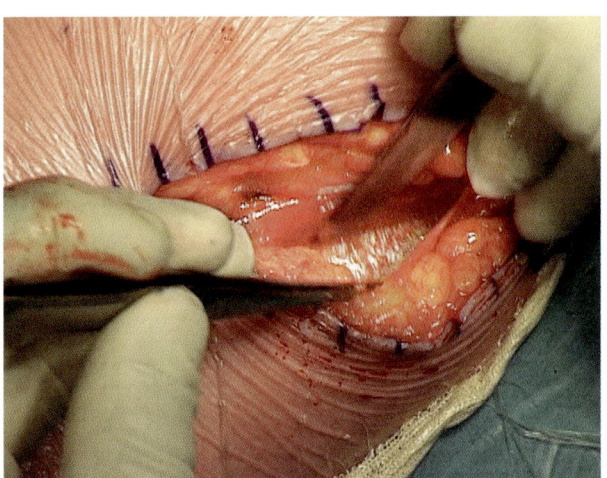

Intermuscular Approach

The tensor fasciae lata is exposed (TFL): its aponeurosis is incised using a scalpel
blade following the direction of the fascial fibres, 5 mm below (Fig. 3.4). The anterior edge of the muscle body is freed using Mayo scissors and then blunt finger
dissection. Once the muscle has been bypassed, we have direct access to the anterior
cervical region.

A modified Charnley frame is placed against the body of the TFL laterally and
on the sartorius medially. One cobra retractor is placed at the superior base of the
neck under the gluteus minimus and a second retractor to retract the distal body of
the TFL out of the surgical field.

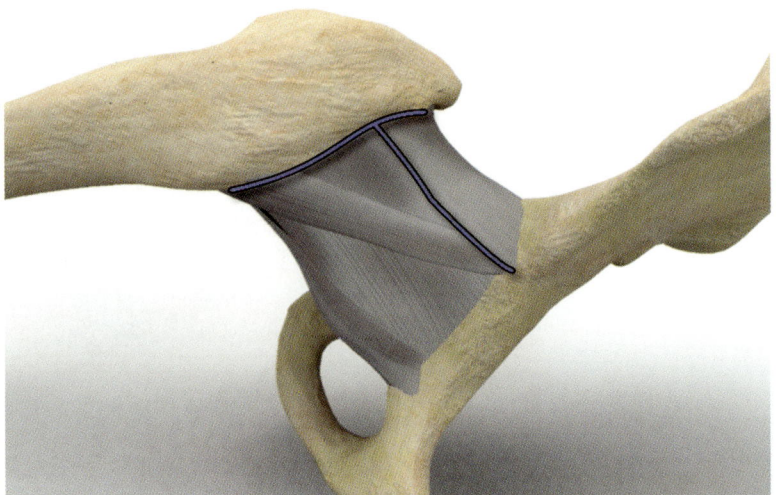

Fig. 3.5 Incision of the anterior capsule

The superficial aponeurosis of the rectus femoris is incised and the muscle body retracted inwards. The deep aponeurosis is then carefully incised and the anterior circumflex pedicle dissected and ligated. The tubercle for the insertion of the vastus lateralis muscle can be seen under its lateral stump; this is an essential landmark for the arthrotomy. Using a periosteal elevator, the capsule is then lifted along a line from the insertion of the rectus femoris to the tubercle of the vastus lateralis, with the limb held in slight rotation and flexion without constraint.

Arthrotomy

The arthrotomy is performed at the superior edge of the neck, from the insertion of the rectus femoris to the tubercle of the vastus lateralis (Fig. 3.5). An initial debridement is performed at the base of the neck towards the lesser trochanter along the inter-trochanteric line to free the large anterior capsular flap, which is preserved. A second debridement is then performed at the base of the neck towards the trochanteric fossa respecting the insertion of the gluteus minimus.

The cobra is then put back between the rim and the apical capsule; a Hohmann retractor is placed between the anterior capsule and the rim. The head of the femur is broadly exposed; the rim is resected using a scalpel blade.

Cervicotomy

A retractor is placed under the neck, with the lower limb slightly flexed with external rotation to expose its anterior aspect as much as possible.

Fig. 3.6 Cervicotomy with
the oscillating saw

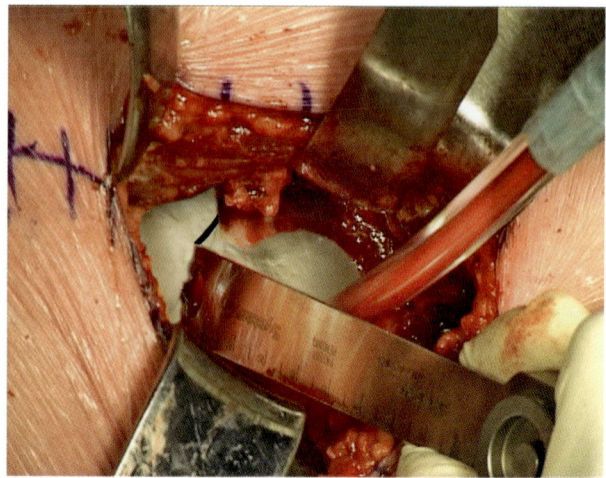

The preoperative landmarks of the length of the lower extremity are transposed
from the vertical axis to the tubercle of the vastus lateralis. The vertical impaction
of a straight chisel, from the base of the neck to the tubercle, enables an appropriate
initial, yet incomplete, vertical cervicotomy without the risk of posterior bleeding.
Motorised section is then performed using a narrow rigid blade, along the plane of
the superior edge of the first prepositioned reamer (Fig. 3.6).

Impaction of the straight chisel in the cervicotomy site enables exposure of the
cervical section via deflexion. A Lambotte lag screw is screwed in the centre of the
head subchondrally; the neck is twisted through 3–4 rotations to avulse the round
ligament. The posterior synovial fringes are cut using a scalpel blade. The head is
then removed and calibrated.

Acetabular Preparation

The lower extremity is repositioned on its supports.

A Steinmann pin is impacted vertically from the roof of the acetabulum pushing
back the anterior edge of the proximal muscle mass of the TFL. The Charnley frame
is repositioned horizontally to rest on the distal body of the muscle. The acetabulum
is then exposed using two Hohmann retractors resting on the anterior and posterior
horns.

The table is lowered.

The residual rim and round ligament are resected, and the transverse ligament is
preserved.

Haemostasis of the obturator is systematic.

Instrumentation of the acetabulum is performed vertically, with reaming at 45°
(Fig. 3.7).

Fig. 3.7 The acetabulum is
prepared with reamer

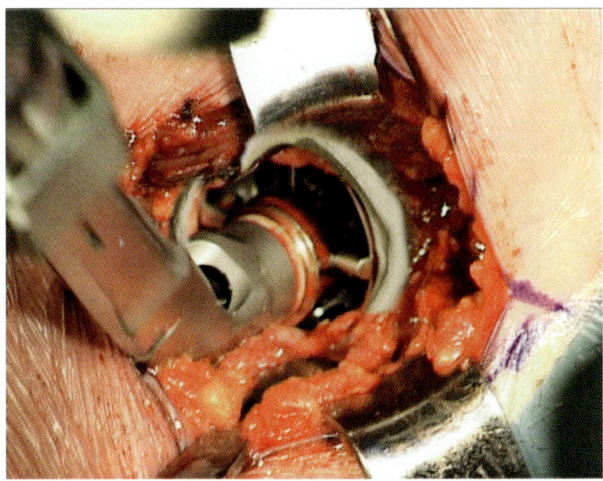

The handle is also angled at 45° and ensures polar pressurisation but with the mediation of the transverse acetabular ligament, thus reproducing the patient's normal anteversion (Fig. 3.8). The exposed subchondral bone must be preserved. The press fit is tested with a trial cup.

The acetabular implant is then impacted using the angled driver.

The verticality indication mark ensures correct positioning at an angle of 45° with respect to the transverse ligament.

Definitive impaction is performed using the spherical PE impactor for a perfect press fit.

The ceramic is carefully lowered using a sucker to the bottom of the cup after lavage.

The margins should be checked prior to impaction (Fig. 3.9).

The various Hohmann and Charnley retractors and the Steinmann pin are removed.

The anaesthetists are asked to check the neuromuscular blockade in athletic patients prior to the next femoral phase.

Femoral Preparation

The table is raised, and the sterile bag is placed.

As with any anterior approach, the neck is exposed by luxation with external rotation, extension, and adduction. In lateral decubitus, the lower extremity is pulled back and naturally stabilised with its own weight and rotated through 90° (Fig. 3.10).

Instrumentation of the femur is performed from the front and not from the side as on an orthopaedic table.

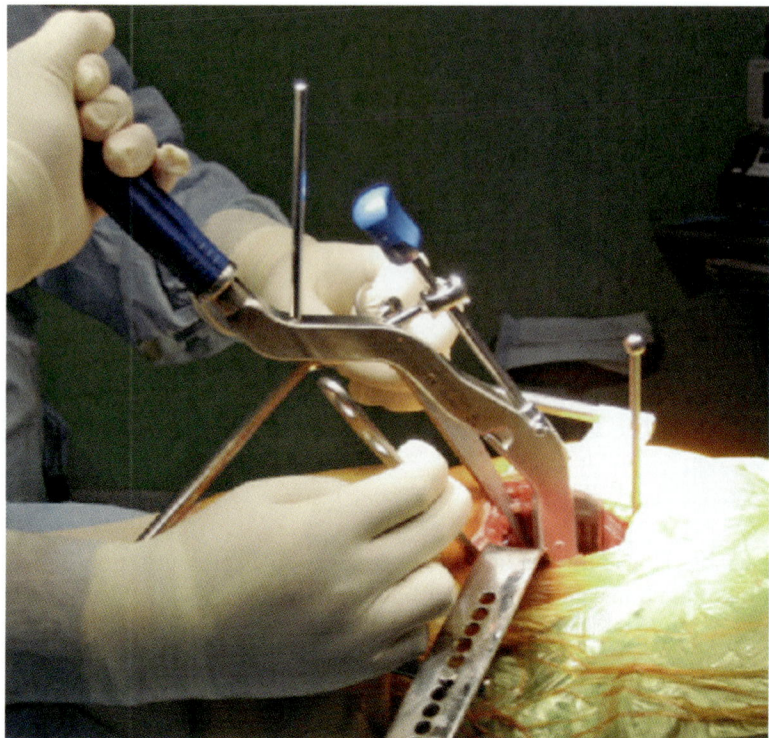

Fig. 3.8 The reamer is angled at 45° and ensures polar pressurisation

Fig. 3.9 The ceramic insert
is placed in the cup using a
sucker

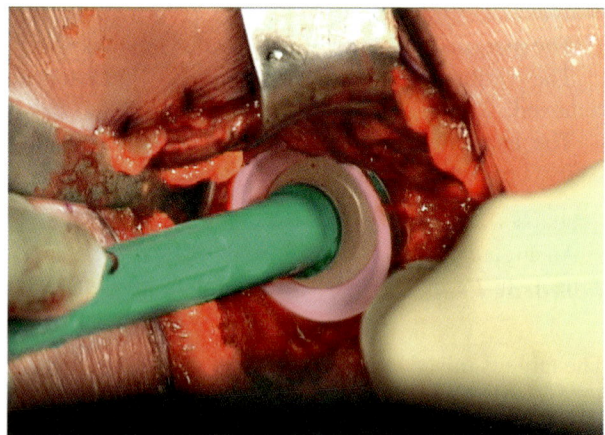

Two retractors are needed to expose the femur.

A first cobra retractor is used to retract the apical capsule which is released at its
base; the retractor is propped against the summit of the greater trochanter in front of

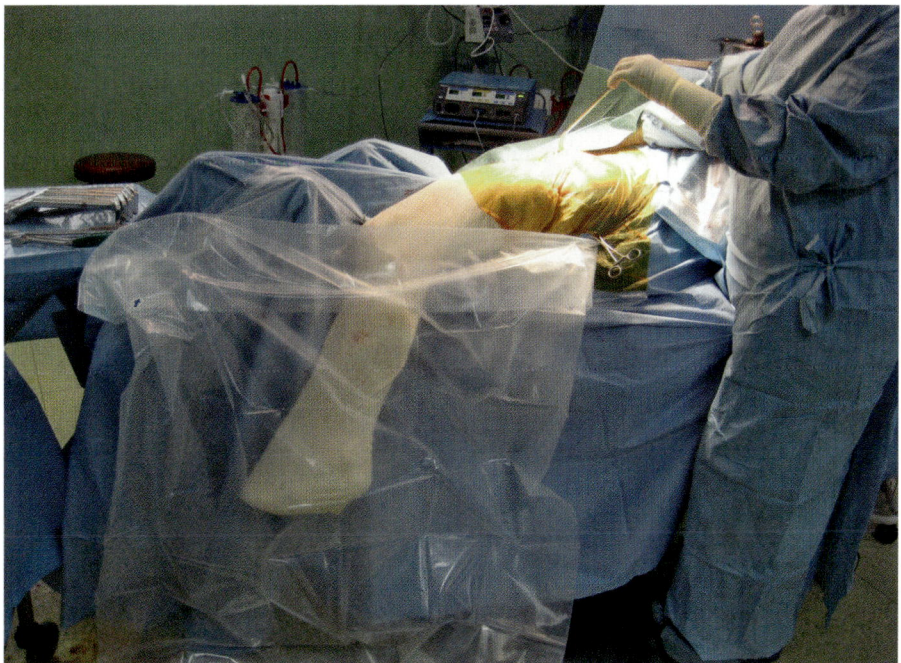

Fig. 3.10 The operated leg is rotated through 90°

the insertion of the gluteus minimus. The second contra-angled retractor is placed against the lesser trochanter and retracts the anterior capsular flap.

The femur is prepared in two phases: cervical and then diaphyseal.

The first cervical plasty is performed in three phases, during which the luxated lower extremity remains self-stabilised without assistance:

- Cervico-trochanteric emptying is performed using an angled punch (Fig. 3.11).
- Centromedullary trepanation requires a rigid tunnelling device introduced on contact with the lateral cortex and then turned forwards 120° before descending and compacting the cancellous bone on the calcar. The suction device can then be inserted to the bottom without the risk of its taking the wrong trajectory.
- An angled starter is then impacted in extension, sparing the anterior aspect of the neck. Its descent over 30 mm prepositions the first reamer.

Diaphyseal Preparation

This is performed in situ, using double-angled 3D monobloc reamers of increasing sizes until rotational stability is achieved. Each time that a reamer is inserted and then withdrawn, the assistant applies slight traction to the lower extremity with 20°

Fig. 3.11 Angled punch is
used to prepare the cervico-
trochanteric section

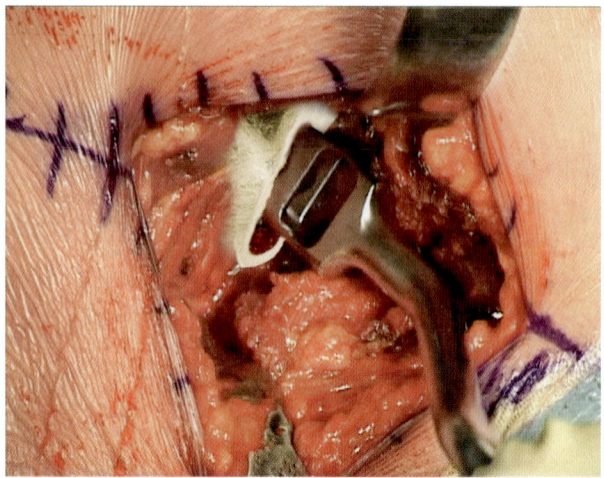

Fig. 3.12 Double-angled 3D
monobloc reamers are used to
prepare the femur

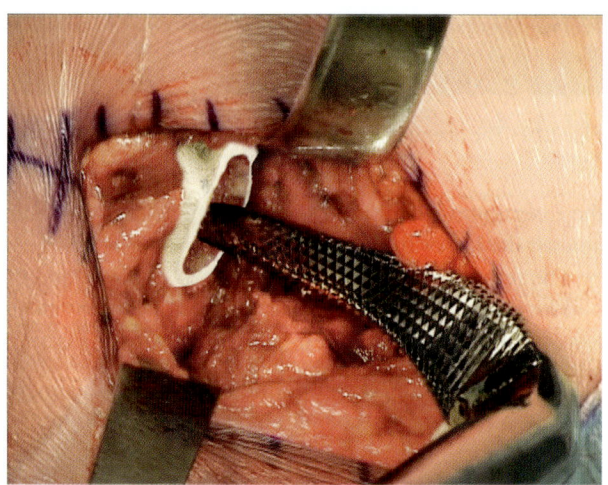

adduction and extension, with constant external rotation at 90° with the limb held
vertical. There is never any fixed rotational stress, notably at the knee, of more than
90° (Fig. 3.12).

The first reamer should descend into the prepared metaphysis with ease, with an
optimal degree of valgus and respecting a triangular-shaped safety margin of cancellous bone at the level of the calcar. The definitive stem is impacted using the
specific 3D implant driver whilst preventing any initial mis-rotation. The anterior
space between a straight stem and the neck is grafted with the previously removed
cancellous bone (Fig. 3.13).

Fig. 3.13 The final femoral implant is impacted using specific implant driver

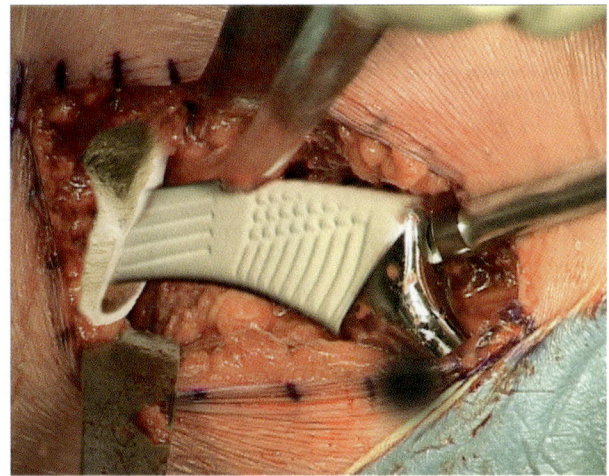

Fig. 3.14 The chosen ceramic head is placed on the dried morse taper

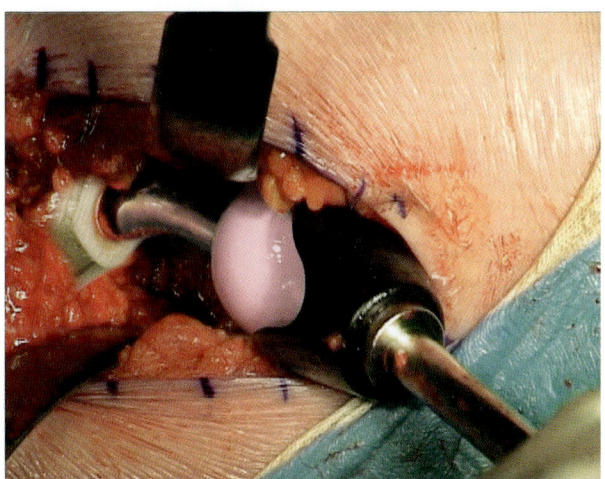

Choosing the Head

A trial head is placed on the definitive implant and enables all length and stability tests in the extreme sectors of flexion, extension, and rotation. It is preferable to perform the test on the implant rather than on the last reamer whose positioning is sometimes slightly different.

The chosen ceramic head is then placed on the dried morse taper and then impacted after slight rotation for safety (Fig. 3.14).

The acetabulum is thoroughly flushed and the hip reduced, the lower extremity resting on its two supports. The Ortolani test is usually performed but not very reliable in patients under neuromuscular blockade. However, its absence is a sign of elongation.

Fig. 3.15 The large anterior capsule flap is replaced and sutured to the apical capsule with rotation

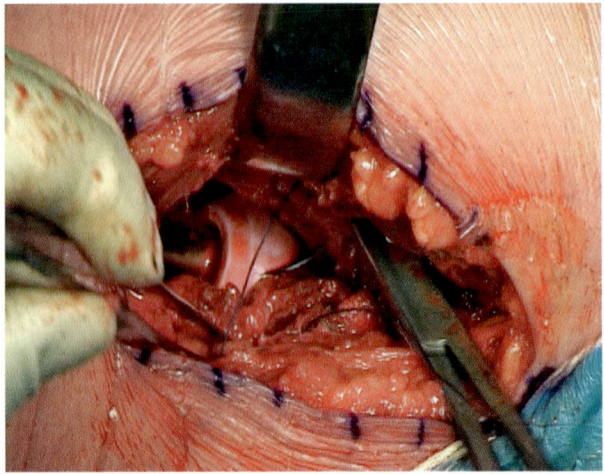

Fig. 3.16 Skin closure can be made either with staples or Vicryl* rapide

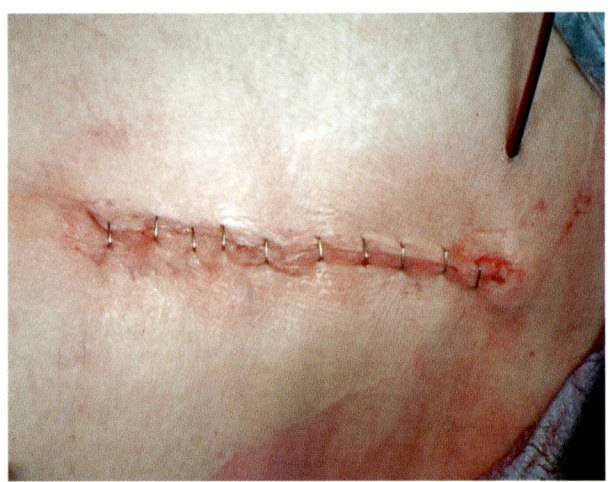

Closure

The cobra is repositioned outside the joint capsule on the roof of the acetabulum, and the hip is lavaged again (Fig. 3.15).

The large anterior capsule flap is replaced. It is sutured to the apical capsule with rotation (external or internal). A plasty may be required to put it back under tension in cases of coxa magna.

If the required length modification is not achieved, the base of the released capsule is returned to the anterior inter-trochanteric line.

A Redon drain is placed for 48 h in front of the capsule.

Closure of the superficial planes is quick: Vicryl* 1 simple continuous suture on the thin aponeurosis of the TFL from bottom to top, a second simple continuous line in the deep dermis from top to bottom, and simple interrupted intradermal sutures using Vicryl* 0. Staples or resorbable Vicryl* on the skin (Fig. 3.16).

Postoperative Guidelines

The patient should be able to walk the next day with complete immediate weight-bearing. This is usually achieved without crutches before discharge, on the fifth day, given the low limits of hospitalisation.

The use of two forearm crutches is advisable for all outdoor walking for the first 10 days, before the use of a single contralateral crutch until D21.

Anticoagulation should be systematically administered for 4 weeks.

Results

In 2.5 years, over 350 first-intention THRs have been performed via the anterior approach in strict lateral decubitus on a conventional table with no patient selection criteria. Surgical time has been between 35 and 90 min, with systematic cell saver. Ninety five percent were given a straight stem and 5 % a short anatomical stem with dual surface coating, all with a ceramic coupling.

The quality of early results is common to all mini-invasive anterior approaches, with a Merle d'Aubigné-Postel score of over 90 % at 3 months.

We have not observed any luxations, but ten comminuted fractures of the trochanteric mass that were either neglected or cerclaged, one diaphyseal fracture on a small dysplastic femur repaired via conversion of the approach in the same surgical period, one posterior incorrect trajectory, and three cases of sepsis.

Discussion

Lateral decubitus is useful in obese patients, the abdominal apron being kept at a distance from the incision. Exposure of the acetabulum is better than via the de Roettinger approach, the approach being offset towards the base of 2TD. We have never reported any cases of acetabular misalignment. The vertical ancillary instrument enables reproducible positioning with a horizontal inclination of 45°, as a function of the patient's anteversion, irrespective of the depth of the acetabulum. No cases of excessive verticalisation or anteversion of the implant have been reported unlike with dorsal decubitus positioning on an orthopaedic table. It is not a good idea to increase the size of the head; the smallest cup available should be selected given the preservation of the anterior capsular plane.

In situ femoral preparation does involves fewer constraints in terms of exposure given the 3D reamers, but it is important to check the neuromuscular blockade of the TFL in athletes. This is the delicate phase at the beginning of the surgery. The cervicoplasty should be rigorous before descending the first reamers. Lateral emptying at the cervico-trochanteric junction is essential; gentle and complete canalisation of the diaphysis is also essential. A smaller pivot than that planned for in the preoperative phase is suggestive of misalignment in varus, too large a size, and possible posterior wrong trajectory. Proximal femoral lesions, which we primarily encountered early on in our experience, are a reflection of inadequate release of the apical capsule towards the fossa and occur during the luxation phase. Extra care should be taken with cases of coxa vara, short necks, and supra-physiological osteoporosis. Posterior capsular release respecting the pyramidal may prove necessary in some cases.

The anterior capsular plane is always preserved, guaranteeing postoperative proprioception. This series comprises a small number of short anatomical stems with sagittal curvature that are particularly adapted to this approach.

Conclusion

The anterior approach is the only atraumatic approach for prosthetic arthroplasty of the hip without tendon or muscle section, in an interneural space, far from the gluteus medius.

Being mini-invasive, it is quick and results in minimal perioperative bleeding with rapid functional restoration.

- The fact that there is *no need for an orthopaedic table* means that the lower extremity is completely free to be manipulated during the procedure, with no fixed stress, enabling all prosthetic stability tests.
- The *lateral decubitus* positioning enables a lateralised and convertible anterior incision far from any cutaneous or femoral risk, an apical arthrotomy that preserves the anterior capsular plane, and vertical preparation of the acetabulum.

The double-angled 3D monobloc reamers enable femoral instrumentation in situ. It is a reliable and reproducible technique with a reasonably short learning curve.

References

1. Smith-Petersen MN (1949) Approach to an exposure of the hip joint for mold arthroplasty. J Bone Joint Surg Am 31-A(1):40–46
2. Judet J, Judet R (1950) The use of an artificial femoral head for arthroplasty of the hip joint. J Bone Joint Surg Br 32-B(2):166–173
3. Judet J, Judet H (1985) Anterior approach in total hip arthroplasty. Presse Med 14:1031–1034
4. Light TR, Keggi KJ (1980) Anterior approach to hip arthroplasty. Clin Orthop 152:255–260
5. Hamadoughe M, Boutin P, Daussange J et al (2001) Alumina-on-alumina total hip arthroplasty. J Bone Joint Surg Am 84:69–77
6. Siguier T, Siguier M, Brumpt B (2004) Min- incision anterior approach does not increase dislocations rate. A study of 1037 total hip replacements. Clin Orthop 426:164–173
7. Bertin KC, Roettinger KH (2004) Anterolateral mini-incision hip replacement surgery: a modified Watson-Jones approach. Clin Orthop 429:248–255. Review
8. Michel M, Witschger P (2006) Microhip: a minimally invasive procedure for total hip replacement surgery. A modified Smith-Petersen approach. Interact Surg 22:1–5. doi:10.1007/s11610-006-0008-0

Chapter 4
Smith-Petersen Approach and Lateral Position with Mini-Stem

Dominique G. Poitout

Abstract The Smith-Petersen approach permits a less invasive hip arthroplasty by not cutting the surrounding muscles of the hip.

The lateral position of the patient induces an easy exteriorisation of the upper part of the femur.

The use of the mini-stem permits an easy introduction of the stem inside the upper part of the femur.

There are few risks using this type of approach which can be less than 8 cm.

Keywords Total hip arthroplasty • Smith-Petersen approach • Lateral position • Mini-stem

Introduction

The Smith-Petersen approach permits a less invasive hip arthroplasty by not cutting the surrounding muscles of the hip.

The lateral position of the patient induces an easy exteriorisation of the upper part of the femur.

The use of the mini-stem permits an easy introduction of the stem inside the upper part of the femur.

There are few risks using this type of approach which can be less than 8 cm.

D.G. Poitout
Professeur des Universités, Service de chirurgie et de traumatologie,
CHU de Marseille – Hôpital Nord, 13015 Marseille, France
e-mail: dominique.poitout@ap-hm.fr

D.G. Poitout, H. Judet (eds.), *Mini-Invasive Surgery of the Hip*,
DOI 10.1007/978-2-287-79931-0_4, © Springer France 2014

Material and Method

Patient Installation

Before entering the operation theatre, all the hairs are cut off and the skin prepared with Betadine[1] (if no allergy).

The patient is placed in a strict lateral position.

The sacrum is supported posteriorly.

Another support is installed interiorly against the pubis.

The contralateral arm is extended over an armrest, and a silicone pad is placed transversally under the axilla and along the contralateral leg which is also fixed to the table with Elastoplast.

After preparing the surgical field, impervious and strong nonwoven (paper) drapes are placed on the patient.

Two drapes are placed under the limb to be operated on. The first drape is made of plastic, and the second one, made of impervious and strong paper, is fixed transversally with adhesive tape and then extends upwards to cover both aspects of the root of the thigh.

Two lateral drapes cover the sides of the operating table, and one upper drape isolates the patient from the anaesthesiologist.

A limb bag is fixed to the front end of the anterior drape. The operated limb is sheathed in an impervious sock which allows for the free movement of the limb.

An opposite film is applied on the surgical field.

Surgeons Position

The surgeon stands behind the patient; the first assistant stands on the opposite side; a second assistant stands to the right of the surgeon (if the surgery is performed on the left hip) or to the left (if the surgery is performed on the right hip). The second assistant stands between the surgeon and the drapes isolating the patient from the anaesthesiologist.

The scrub nurse stands opposite to the second assistant with the instrument table facing her.

Incision

The incision is marked by a line measuring 8 cm and running at 1 cm in front of the *greater trochanter* and over it. It is slightly curved forward (20°) in its upper portion.

Incision of the skin and subcutaneous tissues is followed by haemostasis.

---

[1] Is an Iodine liquid used to sterilize the skin - Betadine Scrub

Surgical Approach

Opening of the anterior fascia of the *tensor* of the *fascia lata* over 12 cm, following the same direction as the skin incision (2 cm at either sides of the skin incision).

One then sees the anterior border of *gluteus medius* and the superior border of *vastus lateralis*.

In the gap between the two muscles, one finds fat and, along the upper border of the intermuscular triangle, one sees a vessel which must be coagulated.

The anterior hip capsule is approached by retracting the heads of *gluteus medius* and *vastus lateralis* using Farabeuf's retractors. This gives direct access to the anterior aspect of the joint capsule.

The capsule must be cleared of any remaining muscle tissue and fat, using Cauchois chisels.

Two pointed Hohmann bone forceps are inserted under the *gluteus muscles* above and *vastus lateralis* below. One angulated anterior Hohmann retractor is introduced against the antero-superior border of the acetabulum in contact with the bone and under the anterior extension of the muscle.

When introducing this retractor, care must be taken of not damaging the neighboring femoral vessels as well as the *femoral nerve* which is in the vicinity, at about 1 cm medially.

The incision of the joint capsule is made longitudinally and extends over the lateral border of the *greater trochanter* on its superior-anterior 1/3.

The anterior insertions of the capsule are detached.

Make two transverse incisions on the capsule:

- One in contact with the acetabulum, at either sides of the first incision
- The second one laterally, along the lateral insertion of the capsule which has been detached (*gluteus minimus* is situated above and *vastus lateralis* below the insertions to the bone)

Remove the two pointed Hohmann retractors and introduce two Hohmann retractors with a collar under the capsule against the femoral neck.

Femoral Head Section

Identify the *lesser trochanter* with the tip of a finger and cut the femoral neck at 1.5 cm from this landmark; the cut is nearly horizontal (60°). Place the hip in lateral rotation in order to cut the posterior wall of the femoral neck more easily.

Introduce a corkscrew at the cartilage/neck junction. The corkscrew must be inserted horizontally and act as a lever arm between the neck cut and the *greater trochanter*; this allows bringing the head out after transecting the round ligament (if necessary) or after fragmenting the femoral head. A spatula may have to be inserted into the acetabulum to help delivering the head.

After replacing the lateral Hohmann retractors with collars by pointed Hohmann retractors which are impacted into the peri-acetabular bone, introduce a narrow, pointed and angulated Hohmann retractor under the posterior acetabular lunate surface in order to expose the entire acetabular rim.

Acetabular Preparation

Ream the cotyle using reamers of increasing diameters. It is better to use round reamers rather than truncated reamers as the latter tend to produce asymmetric holes.

Ream the socket until reaching well-vascularised, cancellous bone and make sure all the cartilage and subchondral bone has been removed from the acetabular socket.

Insert the trial components to check the size of the cup to be used.

It is important to remove all the posterior osteophytes as they could be responsible for a cam effect and cause the prosthesis to dislocate in lateral rotation.

Fixation of the Prosthetic Cup

Impaction of an acetabular cup coated with porous metal (titanium porous metal back).

The cup must fit snugly into the cavity. If not, try a larger size or continue to ream out the bottom of the cavity using a reamer of a smaller diameter, to dig in the back of the acetabulum.

Introducing and Fixation of the Insert

When introducing the alumina insert, carefully check the whole acetabular rim to make sure it is aligned with the metal backing.

The slightest offset would cause jamming, and it would then be very difficult to remove the insert without removing the whole prosthesis with its metal backing.

After impacting the insert, check that it is stable and correctly positioned (40° horizontally with a maximum of 10° of anteversion). Check the absence of acetabular bone protruding on the posterior aspect.

Remove the retractors and put a sponge impregnated with an iodine-based antiseptic into the acetabulum.

Stem Fixation

Put the lower limb to lateral rotation, perpendicular to the plane of the patient's body and inserted into a sterile bag. The bag is strapped transversally to the surgical drapes.

This manoeuvre allows the tip of the femur to come out of the incision and to expose the neck.

A pointed Hohmann retractor is inserted away from the greater trochanter in order to reflect the *tensor fasciae latae* and place it under the trochanter.

A narrow Hohmann retractor is put into the *round ligament fossa*[2] to spread the anterior bundles of *gluteus minimus* and *gluteus medius* muscles apart.

Trauma to the muscle tissues will be minimised if the initial incision on the greater trochanter is long enough. If it is not the case and if muscles have been damaged, take care of resecting the damaged fibres afterwards.

At this stage, a third pointed, but wider, Hohmann is placed right above the *lesser trochanter*.

Its role is to externalise the femur and push the muscle masses back inside the wound.

After the neck of the femur has been well individualised, the cancellous bone is drilled at the lower medical part of the neck to form a cavity into which the first rasps will be introduced.

If a PROXIMA[3] (DePuy) prosthesis is planned, follow these steps:

- The rasp must be driven in with a "winding" movement. At the end of the driving-in operation, the tip of the rasp should be aligned with the femur or even slightly tipped medially.
- Since rasp N° 1 is wider at it lateral part, its introduction may be facilitated by using the "reaming" rasp to enlarge the point of entry on the posterolateral part of the neck.
- Check the implant position with front X-rays but, more importantly, with lateral X-rays, in order to check the accurate positioning and the correct implant size as predetermined on the preoperative templates.
- When preparing the femoral shaft, keep a maximum medial rotation as the prosthesis is spontaneously in anteversion. If the surgeon is not careful, the anteversion will spontaneously increase because of the femoral neck curvature. This may result in a cam effect produced with the posterior edge of the acetabulum.

Insert with force the largest prosthesis corresponding to the size of the last rasp.

After checking the neck length and the sufficient tensioning of the prosthesis, insert the ceramic head by impaction.

---

[2] Formation of the round ligament piriformis fossa
[3] Is the name of the THP made by DePuy

Prosthesis Coaptation

Remove the sponge form the acetabulum.

Insert the femoral head into the acetabular component.

Place two foam pads under the patient's leg to set it into slight abduction and to distend the gluteus muscles.

Skin Closure

Then suture:

- The articular capsule over the prosthesis
- The lower part of the two *gluteus muscles* tendons to the *greater trochanter* and to the antero-superior head of *vastus lateralis*

Two vacuum drains are placed on the capsule and another one under the external fascia. Broad-spectrum antibiotics are poured directly into the joint. Close the fascia and the subcutaneous tissue with separate stitches and absorbable running suture on the skin.

Perform a front fluoroscopic control.

Discussion

The small incision is enough to have a good sight on the acetabulum and the upper part of the femur.

We have the same possibility of fixation of the cup and of the stern especially in this lateral position.

The respect of the muscle surrounding the hip permit a rapid recover of the functions of the hip.

The patient can walk on it after some days.

Chapter 5
Anterior Approach for Total Hip Arthroplasty: Technique Without Fracture Table

Michael S.H. Kain and Michael Leunig

Abstract *Objective*. To describe the minimally invasive anterior approach for total hip arthroplasty using a standard operating room table and report the short-term outcomes in a series of 128 patients. *Indications*. So-called primary osteoarthritis, rheumatoid arthritis, and degenerative arthritis of the hip. *Contraindications*. Complex primary hips might be avoided, such as hips after prior hip surgery, revision total hip arthroplasty, posterior acetabular deficiency, proximal femoral deformities, or difficult dysplastic cases as a Crowe type 4 deformity. *Surgical Technique*. Through a straight 8–10 cm incision starting 2 cm lateral and distal to the ASIS the fascia of the TFL is opened anteriorly. After obtaining hemostasis, the rectus femoris is identified and retracted medially with or without transecting the indirect head. The gluteus medius and minimus and TFL are retracted laterally to expose the hip capsule. After capsulectomy and femoral neck osteotomy, the acetabulum is exposed. The patients' legs are placed in the figure-of-four position, with the operative hip extended and the femur externally rotated to expose the femoral canal. A press fit or cemented femoral component can be used with this approach. *Postoperative Management*. Postoperatively, hip flexion is limited to 90° for 4 weeks. Patients are encouraged to ambulate on postoperative day 1 and are usually ready for discharge to home by postoperative day 4. *Results*. One hundred and 141 hips were operated on in 128 patients during a 1-year period (2007). There were 26 cemented femoral

M.S.H. Kain, MD
M.E. Müller Foundation North America, Lahey Hospital and Medical Center,
Department of Orthopaedic Surgery, Burlington, MA 01805, USA
e-mail: mshkain@gmail.com

M. Leunig, MD (✉)
Department of Orthopaedic Surgery, Schulthess Clinic,
Lengghalde 2, Zurich 8008, Switzerland

University of Berne,
Berne, Switzerland
e-mail: michael.leunig@kws.ch

stems implanted, and 115 were press fit. All acetabular components were press fit. The mean patient age was 68 years, of which 84 were females and 57 were males. The average operative time ranged from 60 to 75 min. There were three complications: one dislocation (0.7 %) which did not require treatment and two revisions (1.4 %) for a socket fracture after a low velocity trauma and a cup revision for persistent iliopsoas pain. Radiographic evaluation of acetabular cup position demonstrated the median abduction angle of 44° and anteversion of 23°.

Keywords Minimally invasive • Direct anterior approach • Total hip arthroplasty • Technique

Introduction

During the past decade, decreasing the size of the incision and the amount of muscle damage during total hip arthroplasty has become an interest of many arthroplasty surgeons [1–5]. Decreasing the operative time and the number of days in the hospital, along with high patient satisfaction and earlier ambulation, has all been reported benefits from minimally invasive techniques. The essential goal for using a minimally invasive approach is to decrease the amount of muscle damage while still achieving proper implant placement rather than just having a small incision [6]. Multiple minimally invasive techniques have been described ranging from decreasing the size of a standard approach, as in the minimally invasive posterior approach, to the development of new approaches, such as in the two-incision technique [4, 7, 8].

The Smith-Peterson or Hueter approach utilizes the muscular interval between the Sartorius and the tensor fascia lata (TFL) muscles to access the hip joint [9] (Fig. 5.1). The use of this direct anterior approach for total hip arthroplasty was first used by Robert Judet in 1947 [10]. With increased interest in minimally invasive techniques for the implantation of total hip arthroplasty, several authors have reported on their experience with this approach [4, 11, 12]. This approach enables the surgeon to perform a total hip arthroplasty without detaching any muscle from bone and minimizes muscle damage to the gluteus minimus muscle [13].

Most authors using the direct anterior approach describe the technique in conjunction with a special orthopedic table to enable hyperextension and external rotation of the operative leg to improve the exposure for the proximal femur [12, 14, 15]. Another advantage of these orthopedic tables, if desired, is the added option of using intraoperative fluoroscopy to assist in the placement of components [14]. Several studies demonstrate excellent outcomes with this approach, with minimal complications reported. Follow-up studies report that patients are able to ambulate more quickly postoperatively [16] and have dislocation rates less than 1 % [14, 17] with the anterior approach technique. The tables used for this technique can be expensive and may prevent surgeons from adopting this technique because of cost. In this report, we describe the muscle sparing direct anterior approach for total hip arthroplasty using a standard operating room table.

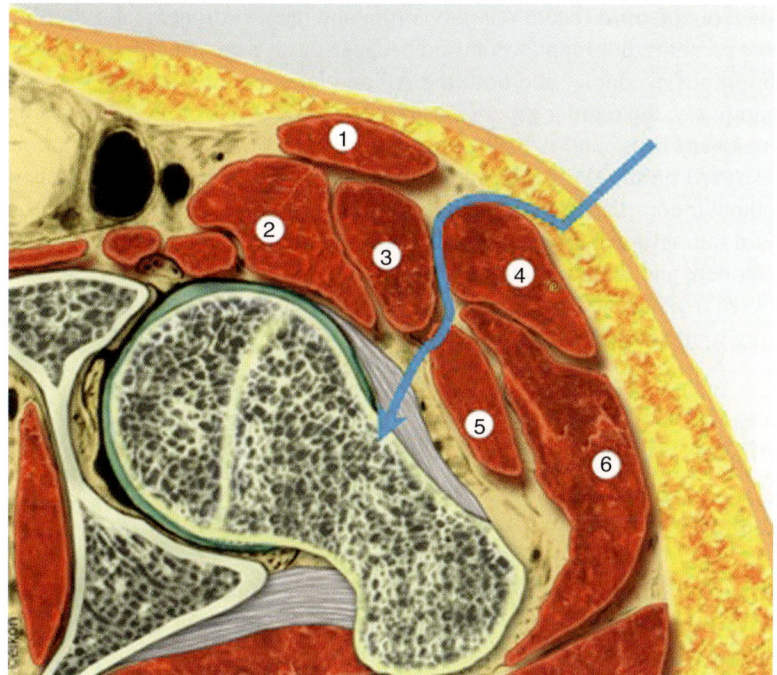

Fig. 5.1 The Smith-Petersen or Hueter approach uses the interval between the TFL (*4*) and the sartorius (*1*). The TFL (*4*) and the abductors, gluteus minimus (*5*), and gluteus medius (*6*) are retracted laterally and the sartorius (*1*), rectus femoris (*3*), and iliopsoas (*2*) are all retracted medially to expose the capsule (*Figure Courtesy of ICON*)

Patients and Methods

Patients

During the calendar year of 2007, from January through December, 141 total hip replacements were performed in 128 patients.

The minimally invasive direct anterior approach was used for all patients. The senior author (ML) performed all procedures at the Schulthess Clinic in Zurich, Switzerland. Two types of acetabular components were used with this approach, the EP-Fit® (Plus Orthopedics Ltd., Rotkreuz, Switzerland) and the Allofit™ (Zimmer, Warsaw, USA). Press fit stems ML-Taper® (Zimmer, Warsaw, USA) and Polarstem® (Plus Orthopedics Ltd., Rotkreuz, Switzerland) as well as cemented stems Weber® (Zimmer, Warsaw, USA) were implanted depending upon the proximal femoral morphology and the patient age. The type of stem used was a clinical decision made by surgeon preference and on a case-to-case basis.

Radiographs were evaluated for acetabular component abduction angle and anteverions as well as for the presence of heterotopic ossification. Measurements were performed on the most recent AP pelvic film and the most recent lateral radiograph. The most recent radiographs were used because these were usually the highest quality radiographs available, and both the AP and lateral were taken on the same day. Postoperatively, the regular practice is to take an AP pelvis or an AP hip radiograph in the recovery room and is of lower quality. Abduction angle or inclination angle was measured on the AP pelvis radiograph, using the tangential to the opening of the acetabular component and an inter-teardrop line. The version was measured on the lateral radiograph between and line marking the anterior opening of the acetabular component and the horizontal line [18]. Both the AP pelvis and the lateral radiograph were used to evaluate for the presence of any heterotopic ossification (HO) according to the Brooker classification [19].

Technique

Positioning

The patient is placed supine on a regular OR table and the ipsilateral arm in placed across the chest and supported by an arm holder. Both lower extremities are fully prepped out with inclusion of the entire lower abdominal quadrant on the operative side to include the ASIS and to ensure accurate assessment of pelvic rotation. The skin is marked to identify the ASIS, the iliac crest, the tip of the greater trochanter and the ipsilateral fibular head (Fig. 5.2).

Incision and Approach

The skin incision is a straight line drawn out starting 2 cm lateral and 1–2 cm distal to the ASIS and directed toward the fibular head on the ipsilateral leg. The location of the incision is chosen to prevent damaging the lateral femoral cutaneous nerve, which is located in the interval between the TFL and the sartorius. The optimal placement of the incision is over the lateral aspect of the tensor fascia lata muscle. Once down to the fascia, it is incised in line with the skin incision. Care should be taken as to not injure the underlying muscle fibers of the TFL. The TFL is peeled off of the intermuscular septum either sharply with a knife or bluntly (Fig. 5.3) until the deep fascia is identified and the muscle belly of the rectus femoris can be recognized. The fascia is incised, and the vessels supplying the TFL pedicle (branches of the lateral circumflex arteries) are identified, ligated with a suture, and divided (Fig. 5.4). These vessels tend to be in the middle of a well-positioned incision. The superior aspect of the rectus muscle is identified. There is usually a layer of fat in this region that covers the lateral aspect of the rectus and lies on top of the capsule. This fat is excised.

At this point, the anterior portion of the capsule should be seen with the rectus muscle medially, the tendon of the reflected head cranially, and the fibers of the

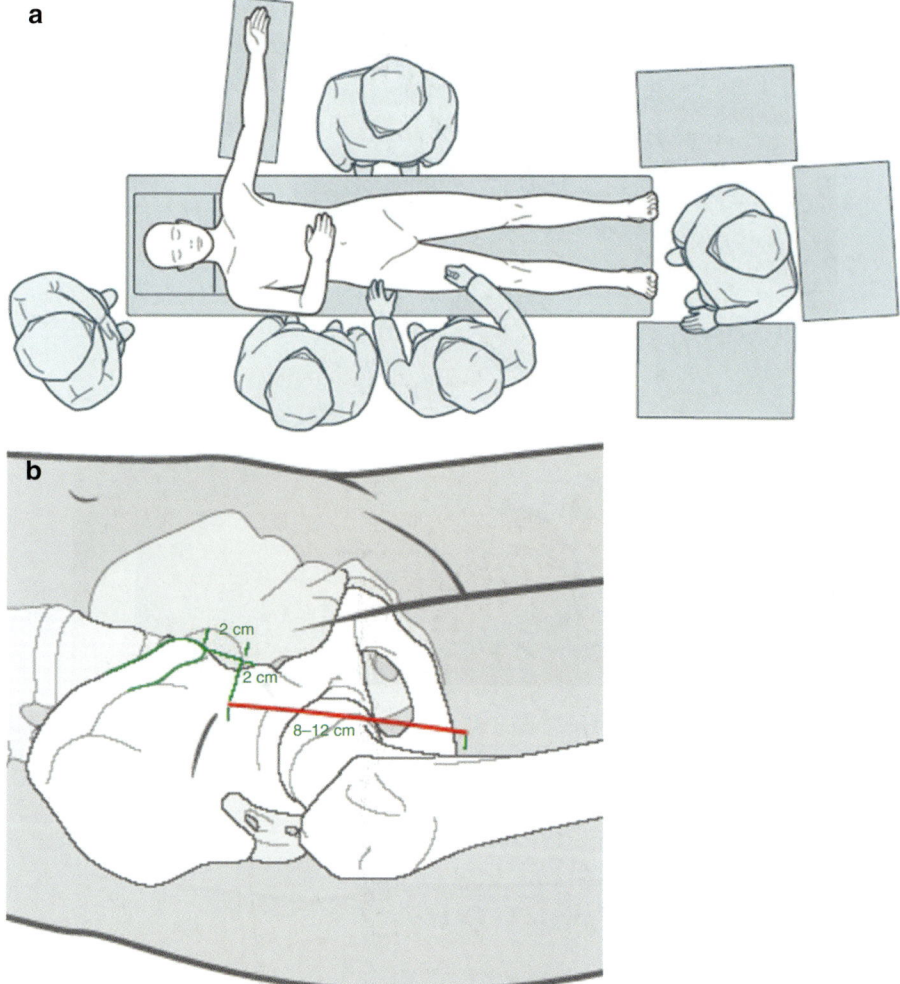

Fig. 5.2 (**a**) The patient is supine on regular OR table. The ipsilateral arm is placed across the patients' chest and held by an arm holder attached to the opposite side of the table. The surgeon stands on the operative side with one assistant and a second assistant is on the contralateral side of the table. (**b**) The skin incision is approximately 8–10 cm starting 2 cm lateral and distal to ASIS and directed toward ipsilateral fibular head

gluteus minimus visible laterally. Distal to the greater trochanter, a curved Hohmann retrator is inserted at the level of the vastus lateralis ridge to allow for further lateral retraction of the TFL. With the use of a Cobb elevator, the plane between the capsule and the minimus is developed taking care not to injure the muscle fibers of the minimus or the TFL (Fig. 5.5). A blunt eva retractor is placed into this interval. The process is repeated anteromedially between the rectus and the capsule. The Cobb should stay along the capsule around the medial aspect of the capsule toward the

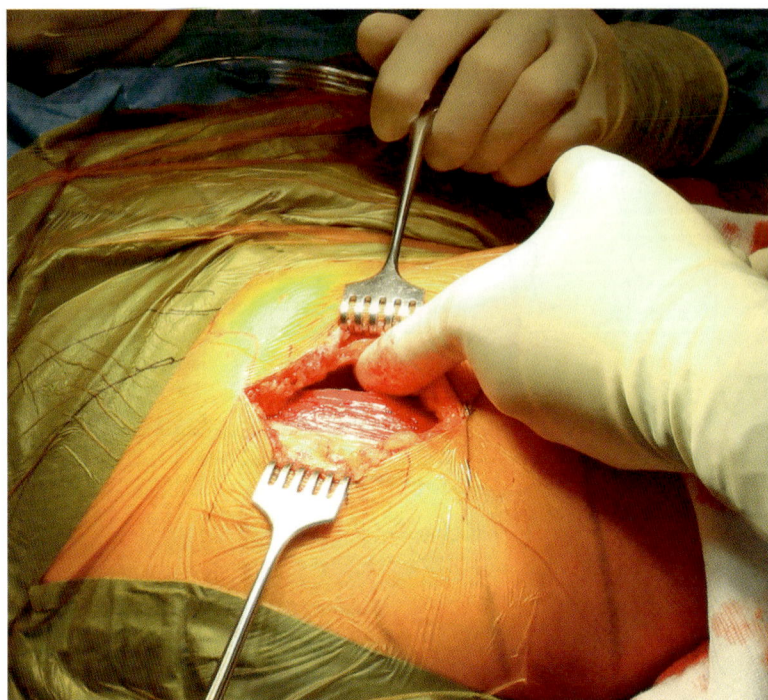

Fig. 5.3 The TFL is peeled off of the intramuscular septum, and the index figure of the surgeon is demonstrating the space between the muscle fibers of the TFL and the intramuscular septum. Langenbeck retractors are placed into this space to expose the rectus femoris muscle and tendon

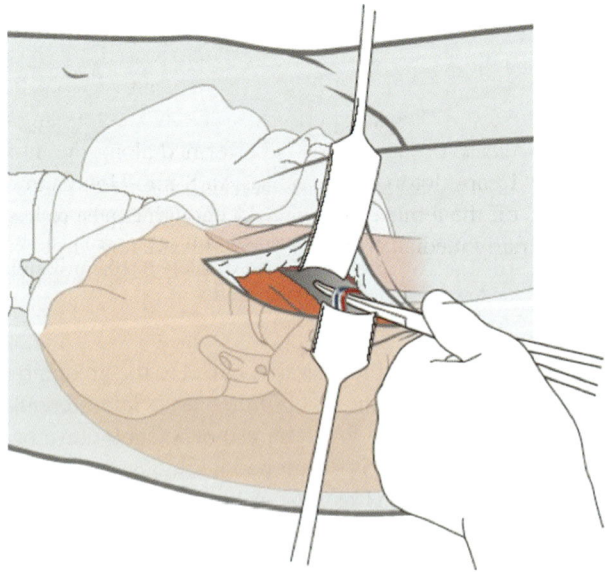

Fig. 5.4 Once the TFL is retracted laterally and the intramuscular septum and sartorios are retracted medially, the pedicle to the TFL from the lateral femoral circumflex vessels is identified in the middle of the wound. The pedicle is dissected out, clamped, and suture ligated

Fig. 5.5 A Cobb elevator is used to separate the gluteus minimus off of the capsule laterally. And anteriorly, the iliacus muscle is separated from the capsule. This maneuver creates space for placement of the eva retractors to expose the capsule prior to making the capsulotomy

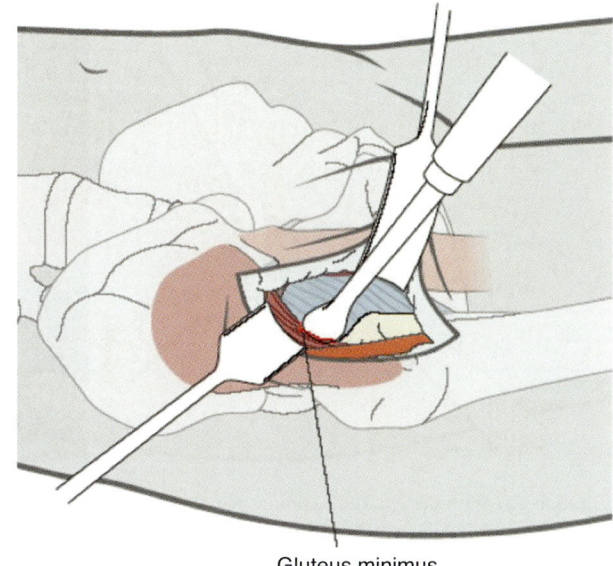

Gluteus minimus

obturator foramen to free the psoas off the capsule. It is important to recognize and palpate the femoral artery medially, and care needs to be taken to prevent injury to the vessel. Again, an eva retractor is placed between the capsule and the rectus and placed into the obturator foramen. Dividing the reflected head of the rectus can be performed at this stage if the patient is very tight and there is poor exposure.

The capsule is then incised parallel to the orientation of the femoral neck to expose the femoral head and neck (Fig. 5.6). This should be performed as lateral as possible to ensure a large anterior capsular flap remains attached to the acetabular rim. This flap is used to protect the rectus from the retractors used to expose the acetabulum. Decreasing excessive damage to the rectus will help prevent heterotopic ossification formation. Once the capsulotomy is performed, the eva rectors are then placed intracapsular, and further release of the capsule is performed along the intertrochanteric ridge forming a reverse T capsulotomy (Fig. 5.6b). An 8-mm Hohmann retractor is used to elevate the capsule off the femoral head. When enough exposure has been created, a corkscrew is placed fairly medially into the femoral head, and large flat freer is placed into the joint to assist in dislocating the femoral head. To ensure an easier removal of the femoral head following the femoral neck osteotomy, the hip is dislocated at this point with an assistant pulling traction and externally rotating the leg, while the surgeon distracts with the cork-screw and uses the freer as a shoehorn to assist in levering out the femoral head (Fig. 5.7). After dislocation, the femoral head is then relocated into the acetabulum. With confirmation of a dislocatable head, the joint is reduced, and the femoral neck is then cut with an oscillating saw (long standard blade) perpendicular to the axis of the femoral neck. If the hip is not able to be dislocated, the femoral head can be removed in a piece meal manner by sectioning the femoral head with an osteotome. This or a wedge osteotomy of the neck is almost never required for delivering the femoral head.

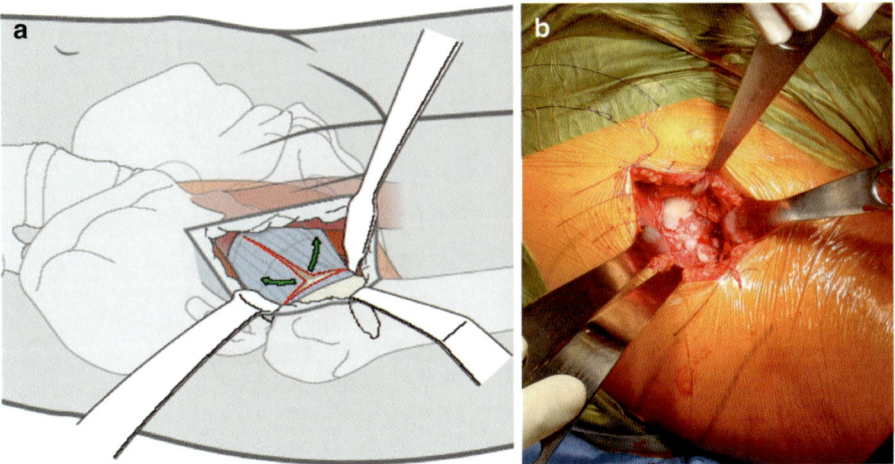

Fig. 5.6 (**a**) With the eva retractors in place, a third rectactor is placed at the level of the vastus ridge. An inverted T-shaped capsulotomy is made, with one limb being in line with the femoral neck and the second along the introchanteric ridge. It is recommended to leave a large flap of capsule on the acetabular side. This is used to protect the rectus from the rectactors, in an effort to help prevent heterotopic ossification. A smaller cuff of capsule is also left on the femoral side allowing for partial closure of the capsulectomy. (**b**) Clinical picture with eva retractors with the capsule exposing the arthritic femoral head

Fig. 5.7 The corkscrew is placed firmly into the femoral head as medial as possible. By dislocating, the femoral head facilitates the removal of the femoral head following femoral neck osteotomy. Often a large flat freer is placed intra-articularly to assist in levering out the femoral head. Additionally an assistant can pull some gentle traction and externally rotate the femur

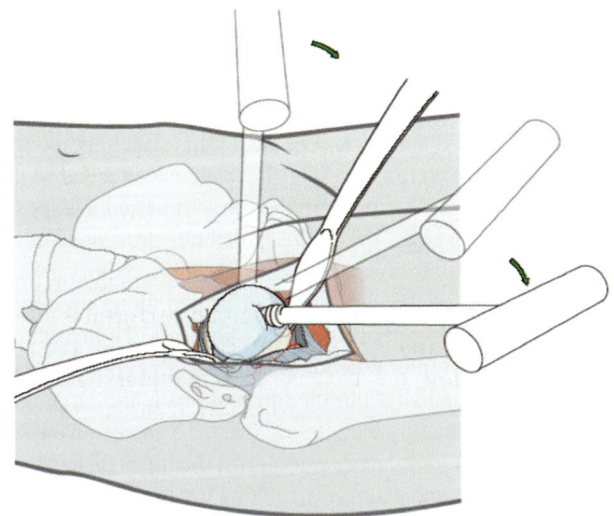

With the femoral head removed, further release of the capsule off of the proximal femur is performed to increase the mobility of the proximal femur. The capsule is also released posteriorly by pulling the femur anteriorly with a bone hook and releasing the posterior attachment of the capsule down to the piriformis fossa (see below for more detail).

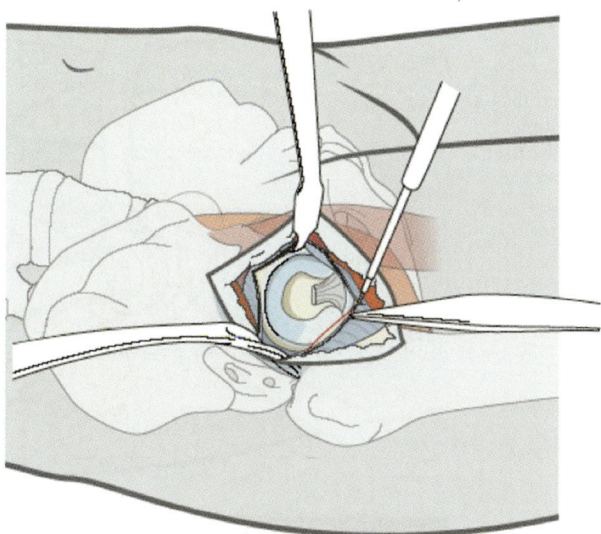

Fig. 5.8 The acetabulum is fully exposed with the placement of two bent Hohmann reactors. Anteriorly, the Hohmann is placed under the remaining capsule and directed toward the AIIS, retracting the sartorius and rectus medially. Posteriorly, the Hohmann is placed behind the posterior wall at approximately the 9 o'clock position. Finally, the inferior aspect of the acetabulum is exposed once a Müller retractor is placed and rectracts the femur posteriorly. Access to the acetabulum is provided and debridement of the labrum and cotyloid fossa can be performed

Acetabular Component Placement

Once the proximal femur is mobilized, the acetabulum is exposed. A small Hohmann retractor is placed intracapsular anteriorly toward the AIIS anteriorly, and a second retractor is placed posteriorly around the posterior wall. Further release of the capsule can be performed after the placement of a femoral or Müller retractor at the inferior aspect of the posterior horn of the acetabulum and below the transverse acetabular ligament. This retracts the femur posteriorly, providing full exposure of the acetabulum and allowing for debridement of the labrum and cotyloid fossa (Fig. 5.8). Anteriorly, a curved sharp retractor at the level of the AIIS is used to visualize the anterior acetabular wall. Posteriorly, a bent sharp retractor is used to allow visualization of the posterior wall.

With the patient in the supine position, the orientation of the pelvis is easily assessed with palpation of the ASIS bilaterally. A double offset reamer is then used to ream the acetabulum (Fig. 5.9). Once the acetabulum is prepared, the surgeon may implant the definitive implant or place a trial implant to assess stability and orientation.

Fig. 5.9 (**a**) A double offset handle is used to introduce the acetabular reamers. This is ergonomically easier than a straight handle. (**b**) Clinical example of the double offset reamer

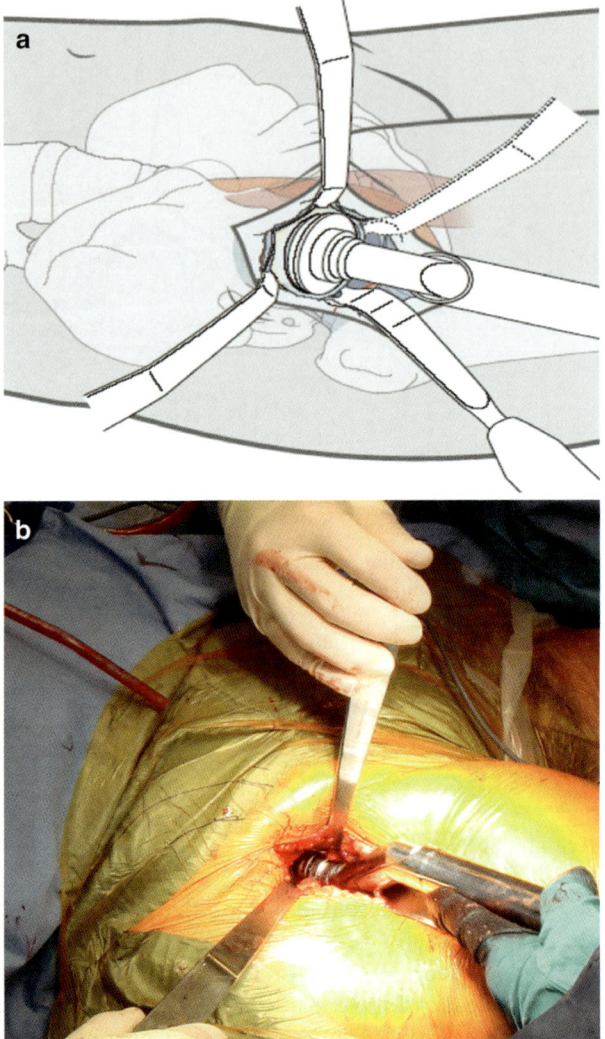

Femoral Component Placement

To prepare the femoral canal, externally rotate the leg and flex the knee to 90° (Fig. 5.10). The anteroinferior capsule is further released off the femur down to the lesser trochanter to assess the length of the femoral neck osteotomy. Separation of the lateral capsule from the gluteus minimus is essential. To fully expose the lateral capsule, the leg is internally rotated with the hip in extension. To allow full hip extension, the leg portion of the bed can additionally be lowered. To further mobilize the femur, a bone hook is used to translate the femur anteriorly (Fig. 5.11). With the leg placed in external rotation, an intracapsular release of the posterior capsule is performed down through the piriformis fossa. If patients are tight or heavy,

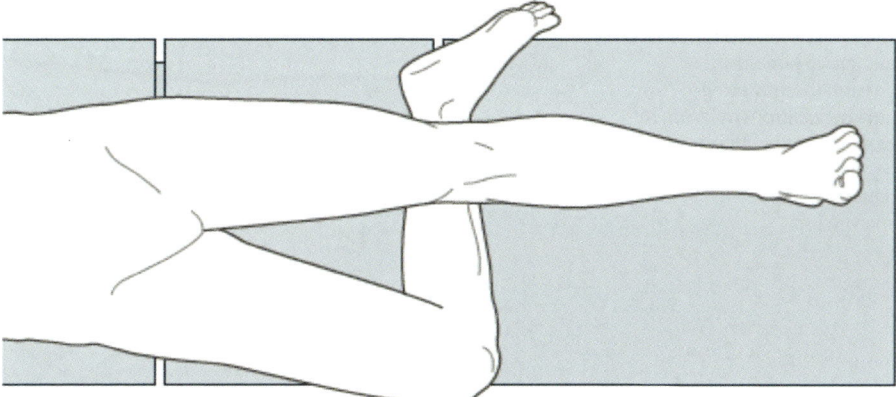

Fig. 5.10 The legs are placed in the figure-of-four position with the operative leg being placed under the contralateral leg. This allows for femoral external rotation and with the foot of the bed lowered also allows for extension of the operative hip. The operative leg can also be adducted to facilitate exposure of the proximal femur

Fig. 5.11 With the use of a bone hook into the osteotomy site of the femoral neck, the femur can be pulled more anteriorly to help put tension on the remaining capsule and further assist in exposing the proximal femur for lateral and posterior capsular release

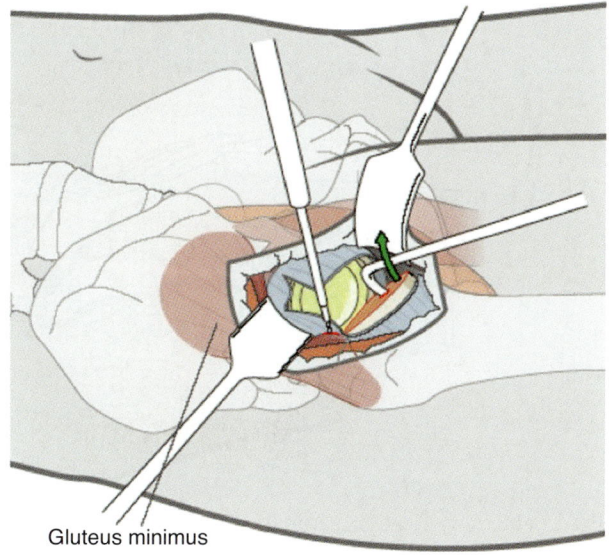

Gluteus minimus

the external rotators can be released if absolutely necessary. To deliver the proximal femur into the wound for reaming and broaching, a trochanteric retractor is placed behind the greater trochanter to elevate the femur and provides access to the femoral canal. To ensure proper version of the femoral implant, the femur is externally rotated 90°, and the knee is then flexed into the figure-of-four position with a bump under the foot of the operative leg.

Depending on the femoral implant, broaching begins. Frequently, a press fit taper lock type of femoral component is used, as the lack of a lateral shoulder

Fig. 5.12 A box cutting chisel or cookie cutter is used to remove bone from proximal femur prior to broaching. Proper placement of the chisel is important because it helps to determine femoral component anteversion

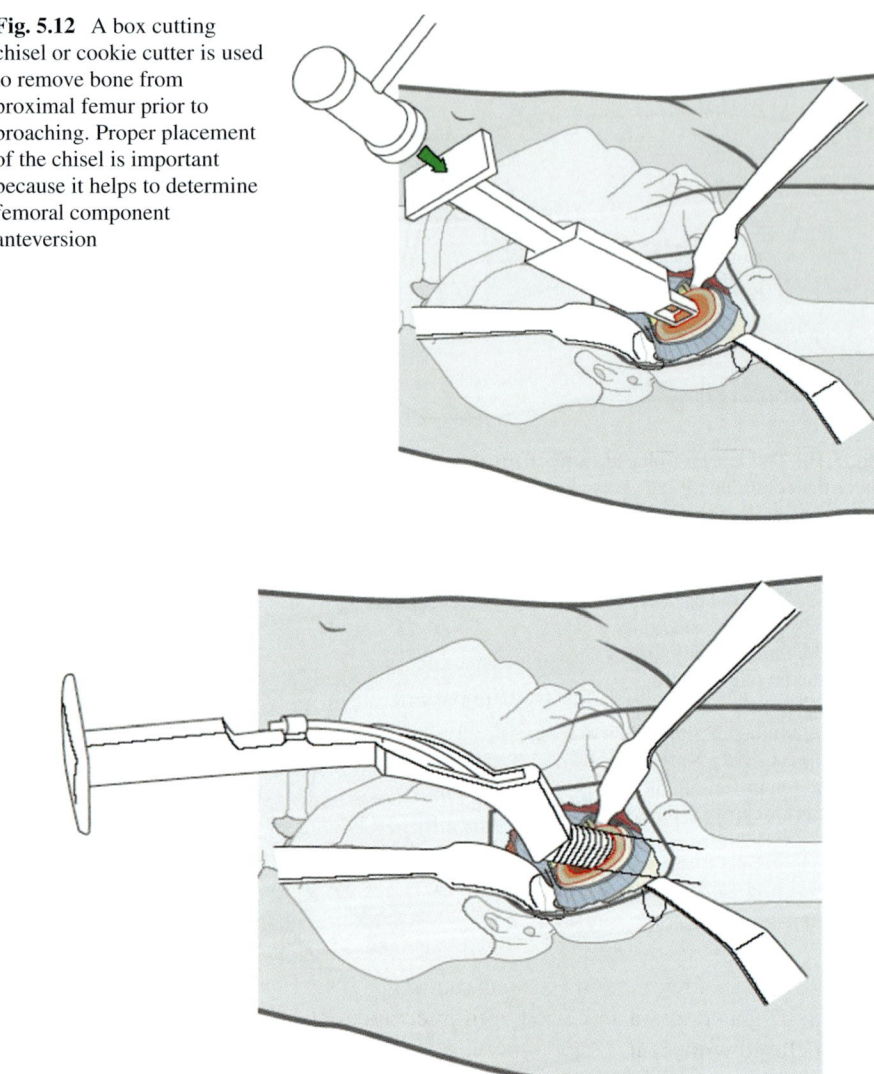

Fig. 5.13 Using an offset handle, broaching is performed up to the templated size. Care is taken to broach enough laterally to prevent placing the femoral component into a varus position

makes this an ideal implant for this approach. In placing such an implant, an offset box chisel is used first to remove bone from the proximal femur, and this helps to determine the anteversion of the stem (Fig. 5.12). To help prevent varus positioning of the femoral component, a rongeur is used to remove bone from the posterolateral corner of the proximal femur. Then, using offset handles, broaching begins until the templated size is obtained (Fig. 5.13). A trial head is placed, and a trial reduction is performed to assess height, stability, and impingement. Additionally,

Fig. 5.14 The remaining capusule is closed. A running suture is then used to close the fascia over the TFL. Interupted sutures are placed into the subcutaneous layer

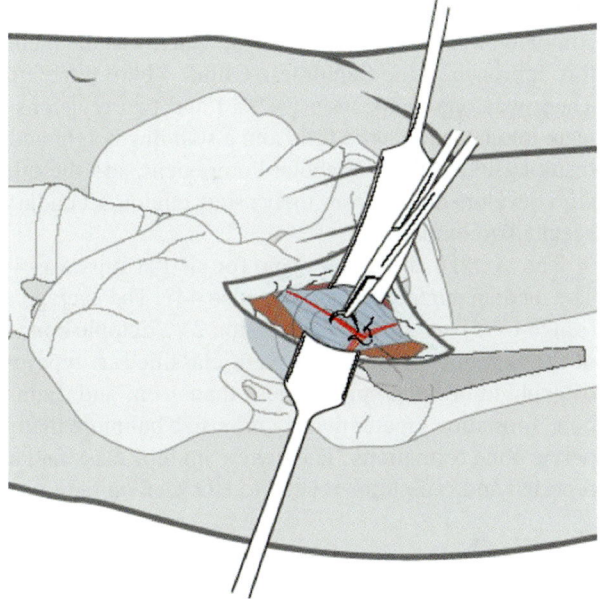

with both legs in the field and with the patient supine, a good clinical assessment of leg length can be performed. Once satisfied, the definitive implant is implanted. Alternatively a cemented stem can also be implanted with this technique. It should also be mentioned that the femoral side can be performed prior to the acetabular side as bleeding from the femoral canal can inhibit visualization of the acetabulum.

Once the components are implanted, the wound is irrigated and a three-layer closure is performed after partial closure of the remaining anterior capsule along the trochanteric ridge.

A drain is then placed in the wound and will remain for 24 h. The fascia of the TFL is then closed with an absorbable running suture (Fig. 5.14). The subcutaneous tissue is irrigated and also closed with interrupted absorbable sutures. Finally, the skin is closed with a running monocryl suture.

Results

During a 1-year time period, 141 hip replacements in 128 patients were performed using the minimally invasive anterior approach. Thirteen (10 %) patients had bilateral total hips performed in a staged procedure with more than 6 weeks between each procedure. There were 84 females and 57 males with a mean age of 68 years (range: 27–90). Both cemented and press fit femoral stems were used with this approach: 26 cemented and 115 press fit stems. Mean operative time ranged around 75 min, and the blood loss ranged around 600 ml (including drain output) per case.

Days in the hospital were decreased to about 2.8 days for minimally invasive patients compared to the average of 6 days, which was the median time for patients without this approach at the Schulthess Clinic. There were a total of three complications. There was one dislocation (0.7 %) and two revisions (1.4 %). The two revisions were in one patient who fell from a standing height and sustained a fractured pelvis resulting in a loose acetabular component, and the other revision was in a patient who developed pain from their psoas tendon secondary to an anteriorly prominent acetabular component.

The average abduction angle for all 141 hips was $44.4° \pm 3.87$ (range $33°-55°$). The median angle recorded was also $44°$. The average anteversion was $22.3° \pm 7.29$ (range 1–35) and the median version $23°$. Ectopic bone formation was seen in a total of 20 patients. Of these, 18 were classified as type one (I) with any presence of osteophyte or bone spicules less than 1 cm and 2 classified as type two (II) with bone formation greater than 1 cm in size but more than 1 cm between the femur and pelvic bone formations. There were no hips classified as type 3 or 4, and no patient reported and symptoms related to HO seen on radiographs.

Discussion

The use of the direct anterior approach to the hip has been used for well over 50 years for total hip arthroplasty and more recently as a minimally invasive approach [4, 10, 12, 14, 16, 17, 20]. This approach is attractive to surgeons because of its use of the intramuscular plane between the TFL and the sartorius as opposed to the transmuscular approaches of the posterior and anterolateral approaches. The posterior approach was developed to improve exposure while eliminating the need for a trochanteric osteotomy, described by Charnely [6]. A disadvantage of this approach is the concern of an increased rate of dislocation. As a result of high dislocation rates, the modified Hardinge approach was developed, and although the posterior structures are spared, the anterior two thirds of the gluteus medius and minimus are taken off of the greater trochanter. This approach has been associated with a persistent limp and weak abductors [14]. To avoid the above problems, some surgeons have adopted the direct anterior approach. Additionally, in the age of minimally invasive total hip arthroplasty, the direct anterior approach provides the most direct route to the hip joint without having to transect any muscles and minimally damages the gluteus minimus [11].

As the techniques of minimally invasive surgery advance more studies are beginning performed to compare the different types of MIS approaches. Nataka, compared the early outcomes following the mini posterior approach and the mini anterior approach and reported that patients with the mini anterior approach had an improved ability to walk at 2 months postoperatively. These patients, on average also left the hospital 8 days before the minimally invasive posterior approach patients [16]. In a recent study, looking at patients' decisions to undergo total hip arthroplasty, the authors report that patients were seeking surgeons who preserved the normal anatomy and associated this with a minimally invasive techniques [11]. It was also felt by patients that 6 months was to long of a time period to recover and it was important for them to return to normal function as quickly as possible [11]. Although, the numbers of patients in both of the above studies is small, these studies seem to reflect current patient expectations. The minimally invasive anterior approach for total hip arthroplasty is a muscle sparing approach that allows for proper component placement and can used to meet the needs of these expectations.

The direct anterior approach can be safely performed with or without the use of a special table. Some authors have described this technique using a standard operating table and reported similar results to those with the table [4]. As a result of decreased muscle damage during surgery, patients are able to ambulate earlier which results in earlier discharges to home from the hospital, and fewer patients require a rehabilitation facility. In the era of minimally invasive surgery and increasing demands from patients to return to normal function faster, the minimally invasive direct anterior approach for total hip arthroplasty is a technique that can be used to help meet these needs.

Conclusion

The minimally invasive anterior approach is an effective technique for total hip arthroplasty allowing for adequate exposure and proper component placement. As opposed to other hip approaches, this is a muscle sparing approach. No muscles or tendons are transected minimizing trauma to the abductor muscle enabling patients to ambulate earlier postoperatively. Many authors describe using the approach with a special orthopedic table. This minimally invasive approach can also be performed safely, on a regular table with the similar results.

Conflict of Interest Each author certifies that he or she has no commercial associations (e.g., consultancies, stock ownership, equity interest, patent/licensing arrangements, etc.) that might pose a conflict of interest in connection with the submitted article.

Each author certifies that his or her institution has approved the human protocol for this investigation, that all investigations were conducted in conformity with ethical principles of research, and that informed consent for participation in the study was obtained.

References

1. Berger RA (2004) Mini-incision total hip replacement using an anterolateral approach: technique and results. Orthop Clin North Am 35:143–151
2. Berry DJ (2005) "Minimally invasive" total hip arthroplasty. J Bone Joint Surg Am 87: 699–700
3. Ciminiello M et al (2006) Total hip arthroplasty: is small incision better? J Arthroplasty 21:484–488

4. Kennon RE et al (2003) Total hip arthroplasty through a minimally invasive anterior surgical approach. J Bone Joint Surg Am 85-A(Suppl 4):39–48
5. Dorr LD et al (2007) Early pain relief and function after posterior minimally invasive and conventional total hip arthroplasty. A prospective, randomized, blinded study. J Bone Joint Surg Am 89:1153–1160
6. Duwelius PJ, Dorr LD (2008) Minimally invasive total hip arthroplasty: an overview of the results. Instr Course Lect 57:215–222
7. Berger RA (2003) Total hip arthroplasty using the minimally invasive two-incision approach. Clin Orthop Relat Res 417:232–241
8. Nakamura S et al (2004) Mini-incision posterior approach for total hip arthroplasty. Int Orthop 28:214–217
9. Smith-Petersen MN (1949) Approach to and exposure of the hip joint for mold arthroplasty. J Bone Joint Surg Am 31A:40–46
10. Judet J, Judet R (1950) The use of an artificial femoral head for arthroplasty of the hip joint. J Bone Joint Surg Br 32-B:166–173
11. Dosanjh S et al (2009) The final straw: a qualitative study to explore patient decisions to undergo total hip arthroplasty. Arch Orthop Trauma Surg 129(6):719–727
12. Paillard P (2007) Hip replacement by a minimal anterior approach. Int Orthop 31(Suppl 1):S13–S15
13. Meneghini RM et al (2006) Muscle damage during MIS total hip arthroplasty: Smith-Petersen versus posterior approach. Clin Orthop Relat Res 453:293–298
14. Matta JM et al (2005) Single-incision anterior approach for total hip arthroplasty on an orthopaedic table. Clin Orthop Relat Res 441:115–124
15. Laude F (2006) Total hip arthroplasty through an anterior Hueter minimally invasive approach. Interact Surg 1:5–11
16. Nakata K et al (2008) A clinical comparative study of the direct anterior with mini-posterior approach two consecutive series. J Arthroplasty 426:698–704
17. Siguier T et al (2004) Mini-incision anterior approach does not increase dislocation rate: a study of 1037 total hip replacements. Clin Orthop Relat Res 426:164–173
18. Woo RY, Morrey BF (1982) Dislocations after total hip arthroplasty. J Bone Joint Surg Am 64:1295–1306
19. Brooker AF et al (1973) Ectopic ossification following total hip replacement. Incidence and a method of classification. J Bone Joint Surg Am 55:1629–1632
20. Rachbauer F (2006) Minimally invasive total hip arthroplasty. Anterior approach. Orthopade 35:723–724, 726–729

Chapter 6
The Anterolateral Watson Jones Approach in Total Hip Replacement in the Supine Position

Pierre Henky

Abstract This is the description of a non-invasive surgical technique using a modified Watson Jones approach in supine position for implanting total hip arthroplasties. The originality of the technique is the orientation of the incision and the use of specially designed rasps. The benefits of the supine position are well demonstrated for positioning the cup in the right orientation with simple and reliable marks. Also, its disadvantages are shown for the preparation of the femoral shaft. The use of special rasps in two parts simplifies this operative time.

We found a very low rate of dislocation and a good positioning of the acetabular cup. The major complication of this approach is the fracture of the great trochanter (0.5 %) that mostly occurs in coxa vara, and two acetabular fractures (0.2 %) with impacted cups. We found femoral stem in varus position in 3 % of the cases.

Keywords Anterolateral approach • Watson jones • Supine position • Non invasive surgical technique

The anterolateral approach to the hip was described by Sir Reginald Watson Jones in 1936 [19] using the interval between the gluteus medius and the tensor fascia lata first described by Sayre in 1894.

This classic approach in total hip replacement has been used for very long before it was superseded by the transgluteal approach (Hardinge type). It has come back into fashion these past few years as it is not much aggressive to the gluteus medius [2, 4].

P. Henky
2a, rue du Grand Couronné, Strasbourg 67000, France
e-mail: piehen@evc.net

D.G. Poitout, H. Judet (eds.), *Mini-Invasive Surgery of the Hip*,
DOI 10.1007/978-2-287-79931-0_6, © Springer France 2014

The purpose of this communication is to present a technical description of the Watson Jones approach in the supine position, before dealing with its benefits and complications, and last with its indications and limitations.

Surgical Technique in the Supine Position

Preoperative planning is very important in this approach and most of all regarding femoral preparation. The level and orientation of the neck osteotomy have to be fixed in relation to the calcar and the junction of the femoral neck into the greater trochanter, so that ideal replacement can be achieved in a neutral or a valgus position. The distance between the internal rim of the neck and the prosthesis is an excellent guide as to the femoral stem position and especially with cemented prostheses (Exeter or Kerboull types).

The patient is easily placed in the supine position, with the buttock on the affected side protruding the edge of the operating table a little (Fig. 6.1).

A classic skin incision [19] is arciform and opened forwards. Beginning 2–3 cm under and external to the anterior superior iliac spine, it extends towards the greater trochanter before it straightens slightly over it and becomes straight and parallel to the femoral shaft (Fig. 6.1).

For our part, we prefer to make an opposite incision on an oblique line curved backwards. Beginning 3–4 cm over and posterior to the greater trochanter, it curves and becomes parallel to the femoral shaft 3 cm under the tip of the greater

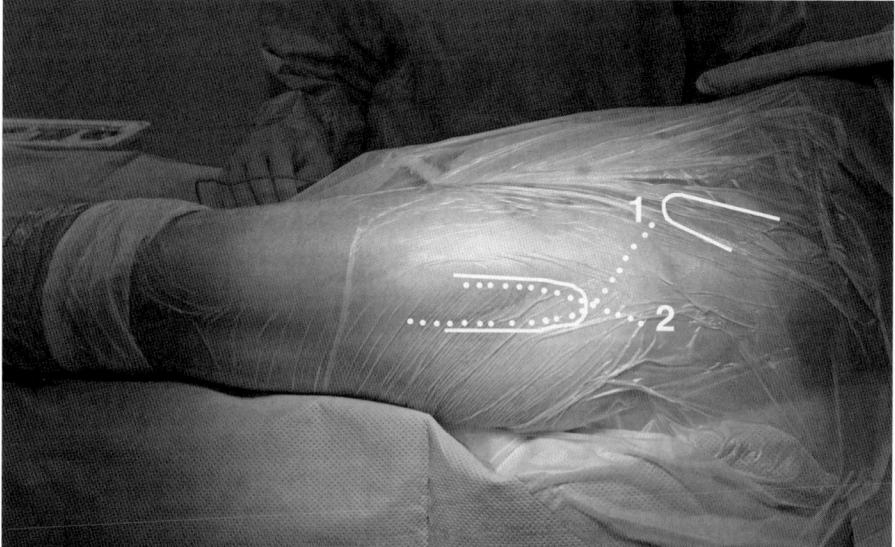

Fig. 6.1 (*1*) Watson Jones incision. (*2*) Modified incision

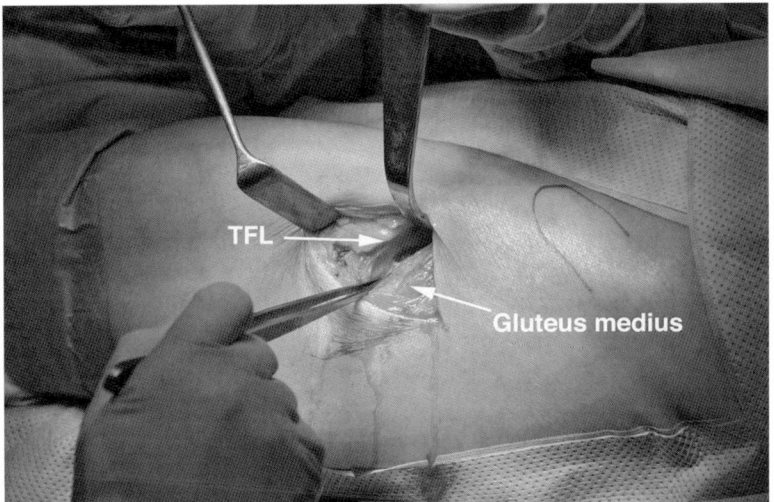

Fig. 6.2   Space between gluteus medius and tensor fascia lata (TFL)

trochanter. This modified approach described by Burwell and Dan [3] authorises a reduced incision length and crossing the gluteus medius allows to find the intermuscular plane easily, with no risk of being lost in or in front of the tensor fascia lata. Femoral exposure is moreover facilitated as the fascia does not bend femoral rotation.

Subcutaneous tissue and fascia are incised in the same line as the skin incision. Then a finger is inserted between the gluteus medius and the tensor fascia lata and the interval between the two muscles can be dissected so as to reveal the articular capsule (Fig. 6.2).

Small Hohmann retractors are placed over the anterior rim of the acetabulum and on both sides of the femoral neck so as to expose the capsule (Fig. 6.3). Once haemostasis is applied to some branches of the lateral circumflex artery, the capsule can be exposed until the acetabular rim is reached. The pedicle of the tensor fascia lata runs close to the ilium at a distance of 3 cm of the crest and it could be damaged if the incision was extended upwards.

The anterior capsule is incised according to an H-shape or in a more simple way excised. This gives an excellent view of the femoral head and neck and allows two separate osteotomies of it, which facilitates extracting the femoral head with a corkscrew. We favour this technique compared to primary dislocation because of a lesser risk of injuring the superior gluteal nerve by stretching [6, 9] (Fig. 6.4).

The first osteotomy is made distally on the intertrochanteric line with taking good care not to take away the tip of the trochanter and also not to leave any superior neck fragment that might interfere with further femoral preparation.

The second osteotomy is made as high as possible, level with the acetabulum. The cylindric neck fragment is removed by introducing a curved Muller osteotome within the distal bone cut.

Fig. 6.3 Exposition of the capsule

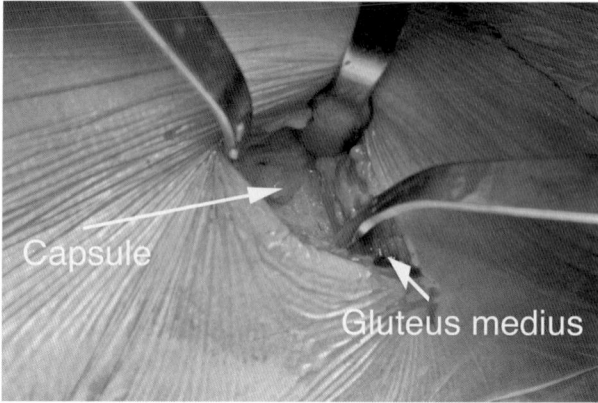

Fig. 6.4 Incision and exposition of the femoral head and neck

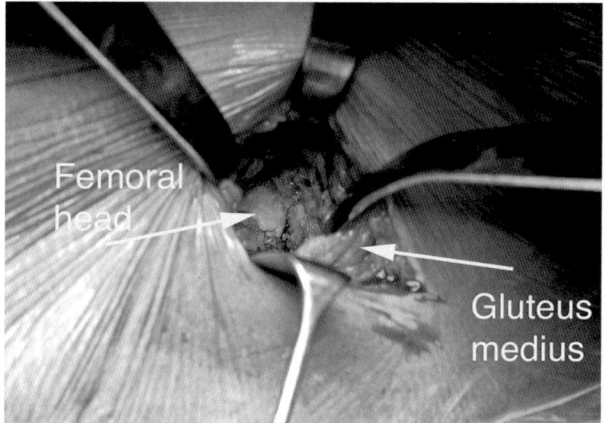

An essential moment for further femoral exposure is releasing the articular capsule. A thin Langenbeck retractor retracts the vastus lateralis muscle and allows to perfectly visualise the internal capsule and the iliofemoral ligament. The limb is then placed in slight adduction, which loosens the iliofemoral ligament and allows it to be progressively released, till the posterior capsule. If necessary, the latter can be incised with low risk on further stability. At this point, the calcar can be palpated very easily and the ultimate neck osteotomy can be performed according to preoperative planning.

The acetabulum is then perfectly exposed by placing three Hohmann retractors around it. The first one lies on its superior rim in line with the femoral neck, the second one is more anterior and the third one posterior with a double curving shape so as to obliterate the femur which is placed in slight adduction. Gentle traction in line may help positioning this retractor (Fig. 6.5).

An advantage of the supine position is that the acetabulum can be prepared using simple and reliable marks, that is to say the edge of the operating table. One only

Fig. 6.5 The acetabulum is
exposed by three Hohmann
retractors

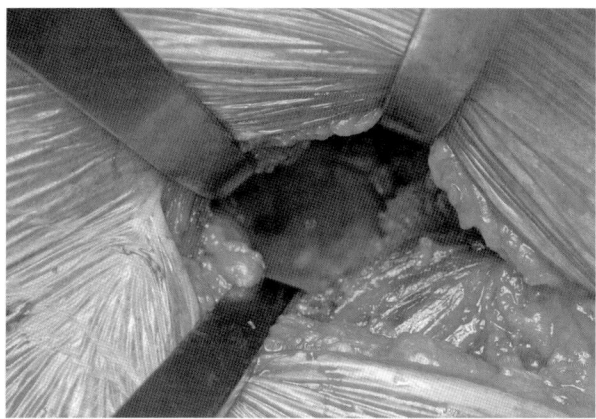

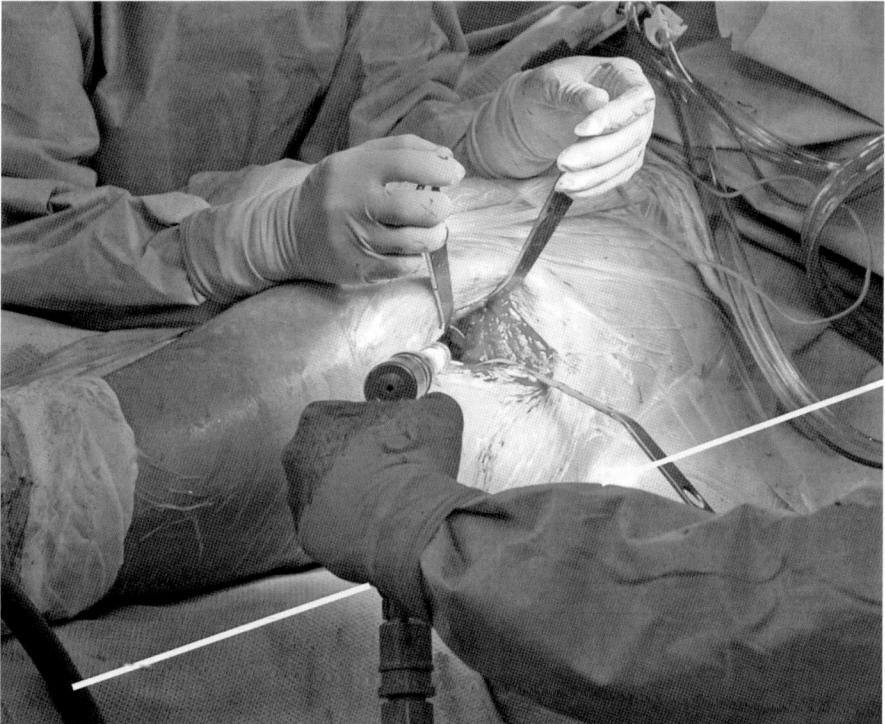

Fig. 6.6 Note the angulation of the reamer in relation to the edge of the table

needs to be inclined to an angle of 40° and anteverted to an angle of 15°–20°
regarding the edge of the table to be in a correct position when reaming as well as
when inserting the acetabulum cup (Fig. 6.6). A cemented cup can be positioned
easily, or a press fit cup impacted.

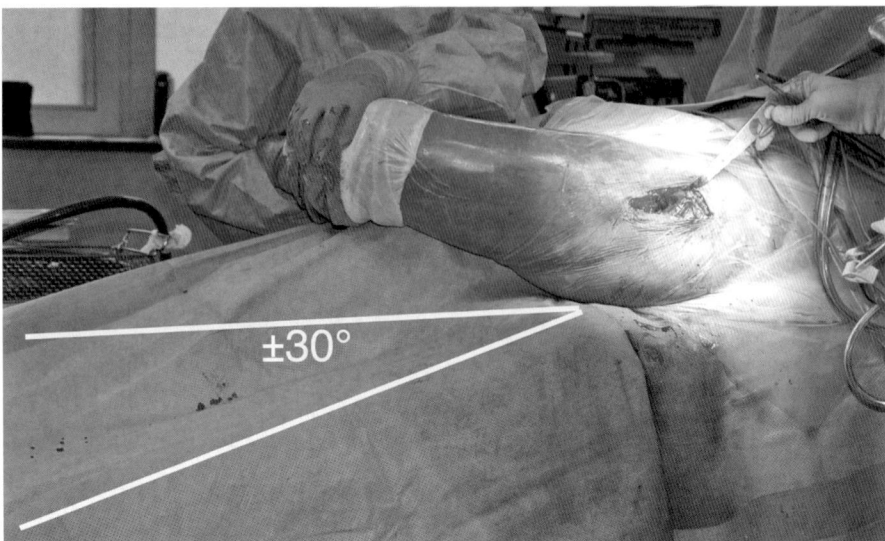

Fig. 6.7 The distal part of the table is lowered and the operated leg is positioned for femoral preparation

Time required for femoral preparation is a main inconvenience regarding the supine position [2]. The affected limb has to be flexed, adducted and externally rotated, with the knee flexed to an angle of 90° and the leg crossing the contralateral limb horizontally, which determines the anteversion given to the neck cut. At the same time, both inferior limbs have to be lowered by letting down the operating table to the level of the pelvis (Fig. 6.6). This levers the femoral bone cut and facilitates exposure as well as preparation of the femoral shaft (Fig. 6.7).

The remaining superior capsule is released and a little Hohmann retractor is placed between the gluteus medius and minimus that obstruct the view and the tip of the greater trochanter. This retractor must not be pulled down forcibly; otherwise, it would section the anterior fasciculus of the gluteus medius. It must be placed laterally so as to unroll this anterior fasciculus which forms the main obstacle to the preparation of the femur (Fig. 6.8). Exposing the neck cut is a more or less easy task; this much depends on the volume, the more or less vertical orientation, the insertion level and the more or less fibrous texture of the gluteus medius muscle.

We use a final device to facilitate femoral preparation. We have had rasps [7] made in two parts that allow to skirt round the gluteus medius if required (Figs. 6.9 and 6.10).

The proximal part of the rasp is introduced in a varus and then in a valgus position passing round the anterior fasciculus of the gluteus medius. Once the proximal lodging has been prepared, the distal rasp that is thinned down and smooth in its proximal portion can come to rest upon the gluteus medius without any injury and

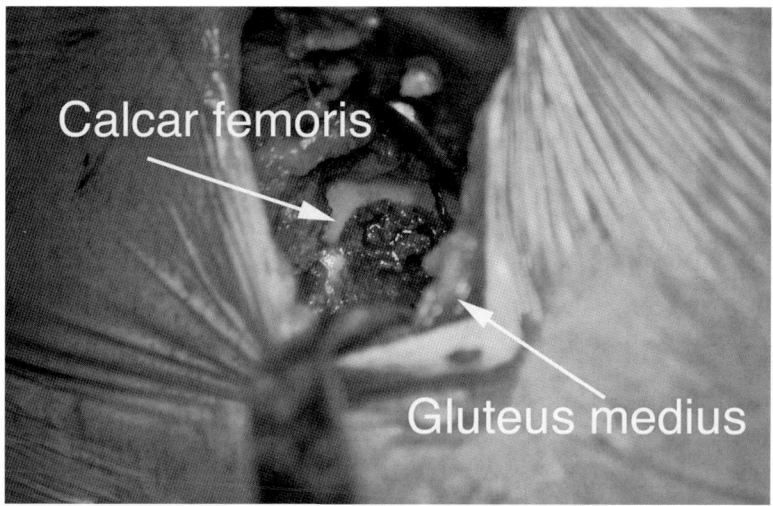

Fig. 6.8 The section of the neck is exposed. Note the lateral position of the retractor placed on the tip of the greater trochanter in order to avoid damaging the anterior part of the gluteus medius

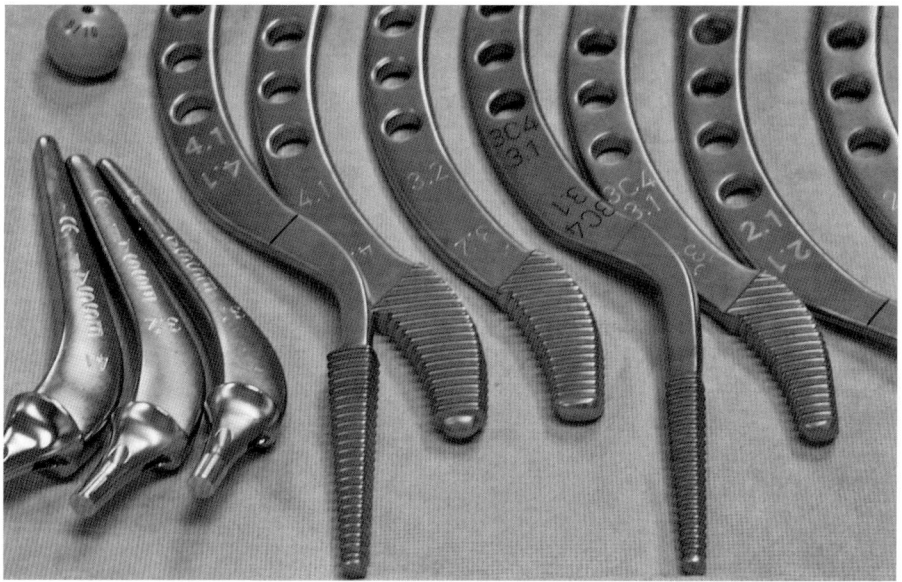

Fig. 6.9 Special rasps in two parts

prepare the distal lodging of the prosthesis (Fig. 6.11). It is worth remembering that tiny lesions of the anterior fasciculus of the gluteus medius muscle are tolerated very well (Fig. 6.12), whereas beyond a certain point, they can induce definitive and irreversible limp.

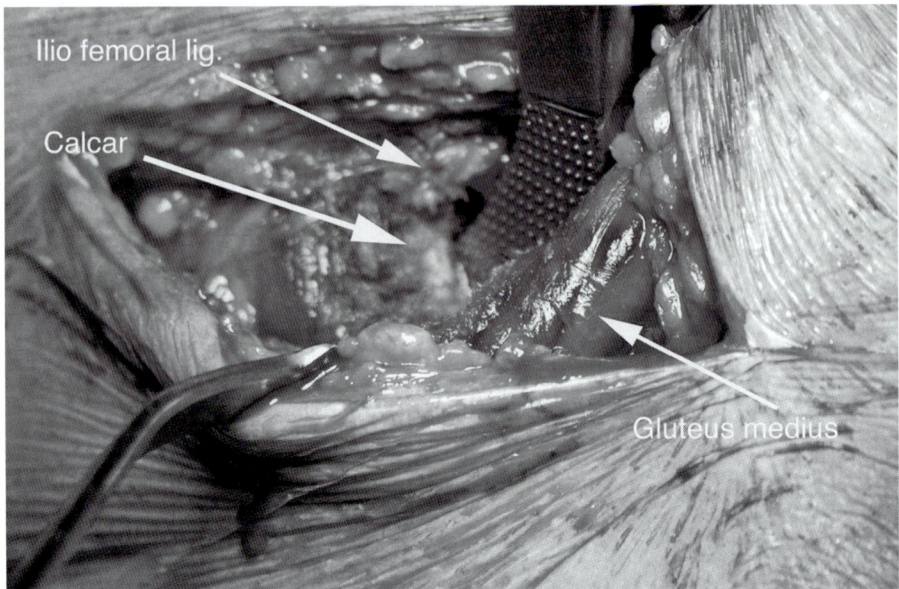

Fig. 6.10 The proximal rasp in varus first and then in valgus. The smooth part pushes on the gluteus medius

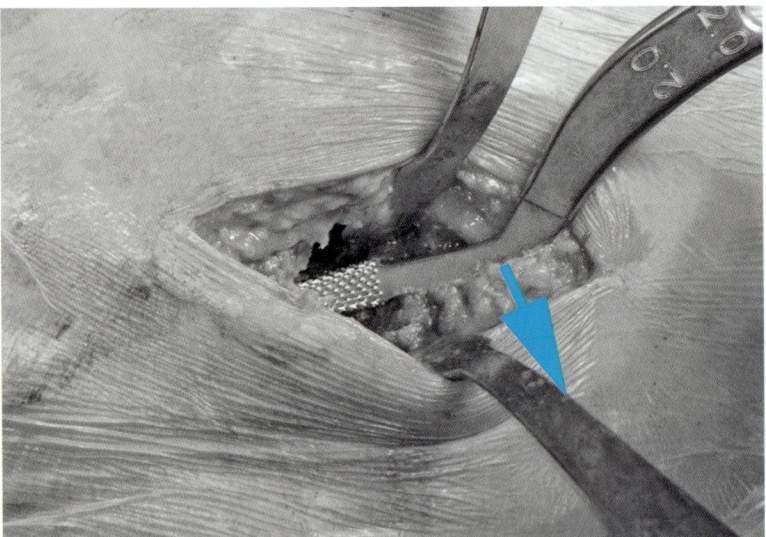

Fig. 6.11 The distal rasp is put into the proximal part of the femur and then pulled down to prepare the distal part of the femur. The smooth part of the rasp pushes on the gluteus medius muscle (*blue arrow*)

Once the femur has been prepared, reducing the provisional prosthesis in the supine position allows an easy measure of leg length, and if necessary, the level of the bone cut or the length of the prosthesis neck can be modified.

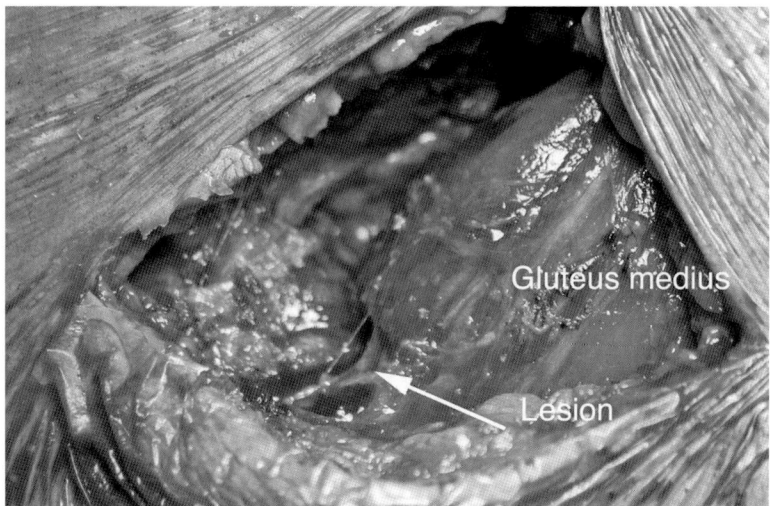

Fig. 6.12 Result of this technique on a big and vertically orientated gluteus medius. This little lesion of G.M. was tolerated well

Advantages

A main benefit with this approach is the quality of the stability that is achieved. Therefore, on reviewing our first 700 cases, we are to deplore a sole late dislocation with a neurological origin, this with 28 mm CrCo heads. This rate is much inferior to literature data that range from 1 to 5 % depending on whether approach. Dennis [5] has analysed the reasons for such dislocations well, and these confirm the lesser incidence of this complication in anterior approaches [14]. For our part, we furthermore have observed a distinct reduced dislocation frequency in comparison with the transgluteal approach, where this complication rated to 1.3 % in our experience. This may be explained because of a preserved transgluteal muscle, a noninjury of the pelvitrochanteric and an accurate positioning of the prosthetic components owing to the supine position.

We also have observed a very small rate of postoperative phlebitis, since the rate of clinical phlebitis that was detected within the first six postoperative weeks was up to 2/700 (0.5 %), without any embolic pneumonia. This clinical rate is probably underestimated, but it is much inferior to what we observed with the transgluteal approach.

This has to be related with the extraordinarily quick walking recovery associated with this approach, which often allows to walk without crutches towards the third postoperative day [1, 2, 4, 14].

The rate of injury to the gluteal nerve also seems to be lowered regarding transmuscular approaches according to literature data [6, 13], and we have observed that 3 months limp, which was sometimes to be seen with the transgluteal approach, had practically disappeared.

On the contrary, we have not observed any significant difference in bleeding between transgluteal and WJ approaches, when retrospectively reviewing two different groups of 99 and 97 patients that could be compared regarding age, BMI and surgery indication. When using the Rosencher et al. [10, 12] criteria, we could calculate a 1,353 ml total blood loss with the transgluteal approach and a 1,333 ml blood loss with the modified Watson Jones approach (average loss in the Rosencher et al. study, 1,944 ml). In the same study, we have observed a significative increase of direct home return (74 % versus 52 %) and a shorter hospital stay (8.9 days versus 13 days) for those patients operated on with the Watson Jones approach. In France, the average duration of hospital stay for this pathology was of 13.8 days in 2004.

Incision length can be reduced to 8–10 cm without great risk, although in our experience, a reduced scar brings no difference whatsoever regarding the swiftness of postoperative recovery or immediate postoperative pain. Its only purpose is therefore of aesthetic concern and it must be reserved to easy cases only.

Lastly, if the gluteus medius is too big and femoral preparation becomes dangerous, this approach can be transformed into a Bauer or a Thomine approach easily [15, 16].

Disadvantages

We deplore a 0.5 % rate (4/700) of fractures of the greater trochanter, which are a complication described with this approach because of the tension exercised by the gluteus medius upon the trochanter during femoral preparation. This type of fracture mostly occurs on a hip presenting a coxa vara with a short femoral neck. Such cases should therefore be proscribed when beginning with this technique.

Because of the obstacle formed by the gluteus medius, the operator naturally tends to have the femoral stem positioned in a varus and in a hyperanteversion position. In 130 cases selected at random, we find a 3.9 % rate of Kerboull-type stems positioned with a varus superior to 3°, which is consistent with literature data about the same type of THR [8]. Good exposure is therefore absolutely required before proceeding with femoral preparation and the inferior limbs have to be lowered correctly. Cementation was never a problem as we had only one case with insufficient cementation and early loosening at the beginning of our experience. Indeed, Kerboull-type prostheses do not require a uniform cement mantle, since they should be closely adapted to the femoral shaft [11].

At the level of the acetabulum, we do not find any positioning defect regarding the inclination which is an average 41.7° (32°–50°). We observed two fractures of the acetabulum (0.3 %) with a press fit impacted component in very osteoporotic women.

Here too, hyperanteversion is however a natural tendency. One has to be careful about it, especially when using metal–metal or ceramic–metal implants; otherwise, consequences may be disastrous. We never used special impactor or reamer for the acetabulum.

Periprosthetic ossification is classically more frequent with anterior approaches [18]. This complication was not a problem in our experience, probably because of a systematic use of a nonsteroidal anti-inflammatory medication for 7 days during the postoperative period and because of muscular preservation due to the use of the special rasps. A shorter use of anti-inflammatory seems to be noneffective [17]. We found no grade 3 or 4 ossifications according to the Brooker grading system.

Finally, we had no neurologic complication in our series.

Limitations and Indications of the Watson Jones Approach

This approach is naturally mini invasive towards muscular and nervous structures [2, 7] because it uses an intermuscular interval where the only risk would be to injure the nerve strand that innervates the tensor fascia lata.

It gives an excellent view of the acetabulum and allows most of the simple moves required there, such as resecting osteophytes from the rim of the acetabulum or making a buttress in case of a dysplasia. On the contrary, it is of difficult use when dealing with congenital hip dislocation in an intermediary or in a high position because of a difficult access to the iliac wing. Also, it has to be restricted to easy secondary replacements with no wide reconstruction of the roof or the anterior rim of the acetabulum.

At a femoral level, it can be used in most cases of first intention, except for coxa vara with a curved femur, where the risk of fracture of the tip of the trochanter is higher. When starting with this technique, such cases are somewhat inadvisable. On the contrary, the Watson Jones approach may be extended downwards easily and it allows any move at the level of the femur, such as wiring. It must however not be used in case of secondary replacements where cement extraction is difficult, because it is not easy to be right in line with the femur through a centromedullar approach and there is an important risk of being misled. But a long external flap may be realised with a preserved transgluteal muscle by getting through the interval between the gluteus medius and the tensor fascia lata at the upper side of the incision.

The Watson Jones approach in the supine position is perfectly anatomical and therefore much unaggressive towards muscular or nervous structures. It allows very quick postoperative recovery comparable to that of the Hueter approach if the gluteus medius muscle has been preserved [1]. It authorises total hip replacements in all standard cases but proves limited in wide acetabular secondary replacements. Major assets of the supine position are that prosthetic implants can be positioned reliably and leg length measured easily. The use of rasps especially designed for this approach and the supine position is of a great help in our daily practice [2].

References

1. Berger RA, Jacobs JJ, Meneghini RM, Della Valle C, Paprosky W, Rosenberg AG (2004) Rapid rehabilitation and recovery with minimally invasive total hip arthroplasty. Clin Orthop Relat Res (429):239–247
2. Bertin KC, Rottinger H (2004) Anterolateral mini-incision hip replacement surgery: a modified Watson-Jones approach. Clin Orthop Relat Res (429):248–255

3. Burwell HN, Dan S (1954) A lateral intermuscular approach to the hip joint for replacement of the femoral head by a prosthesis. J Bone Joint Surg Br 36B(1):104–108

4. Debi R, Bar-Ziv Y, Efrati S, Cohen N, Kardosh R, Halperin N, Segal D (2006) Does minimal invasive THR surgery using the anterolateral approach is the way to go? J Bone Joint Surg Br 88-B(Suppl II):338

5. Dennis D (1998) Review article dislocation following total hip arthroplasty: etiology and management. J Orthop Surg 6:83–93

6. Eksioglu F, Uslu M, Gudemez E, Atik OS, Tekdemir I (2003) Reliability of the safe area for the superior gluteal nerve. Clin Orthop 412:111–116

7. Henky P (2004) Utilisation d'une voie antéro externe modifiée originale dans le cadre de la chirurgie mini invasive des prothèses totales de hanche. 48ème réunion anuelle et 14ème congrès européen de la SOTEST. Besançon

8. Kerboull Luc, Hamadouche M, Courpied JP, Kerboull M (2004) Long-term results of Charnley-Kerboull hip arthroplasty in patients younger than 50 years [section I symposium]. Clin Orthop Relat Res (418):112–118

9. Ramesh M, O'Byrne JM, McCarthy N et al (1996) Damage to the superior gluteal nerve after the Hardinge approach to the hip. J Bone Joint Surg Br 78:903–906

10. Rosencher N, Kerkkamp HE, Macheras G, Munuera LM, Menichella G, Barton DM, Cremers S, Abraham IL, OSTHEO Investigation (2003) Orthopedic Surgery Transfusion Hemoglobin European Overview (OSTHEO) study: blood management in elective knee and hip arthroplasty in Europe. Transfusion 43(4):459–469

11. Sanghrajka A, Mannan K, Caruana J, Higgs D, Blunn GW, Briggs TW (2007) Analysis of cement mantle in relation to surgical approach. J Bone Joint Surg Br 88-B(Suppl III):401

12. Sehat K, Evans R, Newman JH (2001) How much blood is really lost in total knee and hip arthroplasty? European Federation of National Associations of Orthopaedics and Traumatology: Rhodes, Greece – June 1–7: Free Papers: HIP: THR – Technical Aspects II

13. Siebenrock KA, Rosler KM, Gonzalez E, Ganz R (2000) Intraoperative electromyography of the superior gluteal nerve during lateral approach to the hip for arthroplasty: a prospective study of 12 patients. J Arthroplasty 15:867–870

14. Siguier T, Siguier M, Brumpt B (2004) Mini-incision anterior approach does not increase dislocation rate: a study of 1037 total hip replacements. Clin Orthop Relat Res (426): 164–173

15. Siret P, Turpin F, Lambotte JC, Langlais F (1999) Bilan tdm et dynamometrique des muscles gluteaux apres hemimyotomie anterieure (13 cas). CTS and dynamometric evaluation of gluteal muscles after an anterior hemimyotomy approach (review of 13 cases). Revue de chirurgie orthopédique 85:520–525

16. Thomine JM, Duparc F, Dujardin F, Biga N (2003) Abord transglutéal de hanche par hémimyotomie antérieure du gluteus medius, voie de Thomine. Les Annales Orthopédiques de l'Ouest. 35:45–46

17. Van Der Heide HJ, Koorevaar RT, Schreurs BW (1999) Indomethacin for 3 days is not effective as prophylaxis for heterotopic ossification after primary total hip arthroplasty. J Arthroplasty 14:796–799

18. Vastel L (2005) les ossifications péri prothétiques, la complication (un peu trop?) oubliée. Maîtrise Orthopédique 143:181

19. Watson JR (1936) Fractures of the neck of the femur. Br J Surg 23:787

Chapter 7
Transtrochanteric Approach to the Hip

Luc Kerboull, Moussa Hamadouche, and Marcel Kerboull

Abstract   Once used routinely, trochanteric osteotomy in total hip arthroplasty now is usually limited to difficult primary and revision cases. Many variations of the osteotomy and many various techniques for the trochanter reattachment have been described. Our specific surgical technique is presented as well as its advantages and drawbacks. Primary total hip arthroplasty procedures requiring the enhanced exposure provided by trochanteric osteotomy is needed in patients with hip ankylosis or fusion, protrusio acetabuli, proximal femoral deformities, developmental dysplasia, or abductor muscle laxity. Trochanteric osteotomy in revision arthroplasties facilitates the removal of well-fixed femoral components and enhances acetabular exposure. In all cases, trochanteric osteotomy remains useful to preserve the periarticular muscles and to restore the geometry of the artificial hip which are the best ways to prevent dislocation.

Keywords   Approach to the hip • Trochanteric osteotomy • Total hip replacement

The lateral approach to the hip with a trochanteric osteotomy is a very old approach, first described by Leopold OLLIER, 130 years ago. At the beginning, this technique was used by few surgeons, essentially when they performed hip arthrodesis.

In the early 1960s, Charnley [1] decided to use this approach as a routine approach for total hip replacement for two main reasons. First, he wanted to have a broad exposure of the hip to ensure the positioning and the insertion of the implants. Second, he wanted to have the possibility to improve the abductor function by reattaching the trochanter laterally and distally.

L. Kerboull (✉) • M. Hamadouche • M. Kerboull
Marcel Kerboull Institute,
2A Avenue de Ségur, Paris 75007, France
e-mail: luc.kerboull@gmail.com

D.G. Poitout, H. Judet (eds.), *Mini-Invasive Surgery of the Hip*,
DOI 10.1007/978-2-287-79931-0_7, © Springer France 2014

With time, many modifications of the original technique have been made [2]. The position on the operative table has been supine or lateral. Various skin incisions have been used as U-shaped, triradiated, or direct lateral incision. The trochanter has been divided through a plane or a biplane osteotomy. Some authors recommended to maintain continuity between the greater trochanter and the vastus lateralis muscle [3], thereby preventing the gross displacement of the greater trochanter and preserving the branches of the lateral circumflex vessels to it. Anterior trochanteric slide osteotomy, associated with splitting of the anterior part of the gluteus medius, has also been proposed as a good alternative to avoid the complications of the conventional osteotomy [4]. Various tools have been used to perform the osteotomy as Gigli saw, oscillating saw, or osteotome. At last, a large number of techniques and devices have been used to reattach the great trochanter [5].

Although in 2013 most orthopedic surgeons have given it up, we still used routinely the transtrochanteric approach in almost all the difficult cases. After a complete description of our technique [6], we will argue our choice.

Surgical Technique

The patient is settled on the operative table in an exact and stable lateral decubitus position. This is achieved with four special supports used to fix the pelvis anteriorly and posteriorly and to hold the leg. These supports must be positioned by the surgeon himself. It is very important to check that the pelvis is firmly fixed to avoid its anterior tilt when the hip is dislocated. In this case, the pelvis will no longer remain in a vertical plane while the cup is being cemented, and then there is a risk for the cup to be retroverted. Similarly, a fixed flexion deformity of the opposite hip may produce an accentuated spine lordosis that also may lead to an incorrect orientation of the cup.

Skin incision is centered on the trochanter, straight, or slightly curved to the rear to follow the direction of the gluteus maximus fibers. It must not be displaced anteriorly as this would cause the posterior margin of the wound to partly obscure the hip in the dislocated position. The aponeurosis is opened and the fibers of the gluteus maximus are spitted. The trochanteric region is exposed and the trochanteric burse is resected if it is inflammatory. The angle between the anterior margin of the gluteus medius and the vastus lateralis is dissected, and a retractor is inserted into the gap. On the posterior aspect of the trochanter, the insertion of the quadratus femoris is exposed. The location of the sciatic nerve is identified if it is at the least risk, for instance, when a dislocated hip has to be repositioned distally or if the hip is preoperatively fixed in an external rotation position. However, it is not essential to visualize the sciatic nerve if one is sure that it will be away from the operative field.

After exposure of the trochanteric region and checking of the location of the sciatic nerve, the trochanter is cut with a wide osteotome.

The starting position of the osteotome is about 1 cm below the vastus lateralis tubercle which is exposed through the release of the proximal portion of the muscle. The osteotome is directed obliquely towards the superior basis of the neck. It cuts

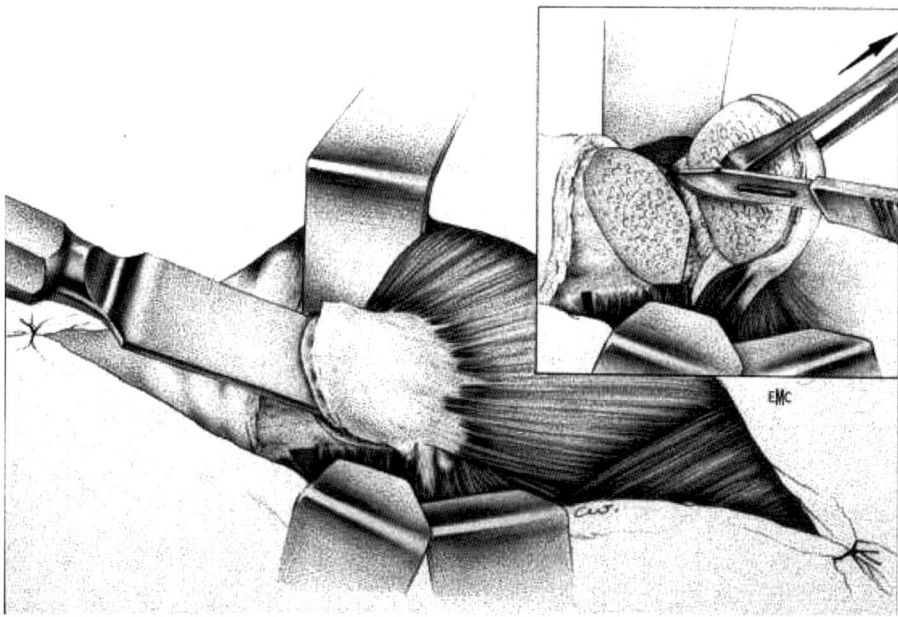

Fig. 7.1 The osteotomy is performed with a bone osteotome following the quadratus femoris insertion at the posterior side and the vastus lateralis insertion under the gluteus minimus at the anterior side

the anterior cortex between the vastus and gluteus minimus insertions, the posterior cortex just above the quadratus femoris (Fig. 7.1), so that all the gluteus medius and minimus as well as the external rotators, but the quadratus femoris, remain attached to the trochanter fragment.

A plane section is preferred to allow the trochanter to be reattached in the best position in order to restore the balance of abductor and external rotator muscles and if necessary to improve the lever arm of the abductor muscles.

The trochanter is progressively elevated with a retractor, whereas the fibers of the gluteus minimus are separated from the capsule with a scalpel (Fig. 7.2).

The trochanter with muscles attached to it is maintained with two or three pins above the superior and posterior rim of the acetabulum, posteriorly because the external obturator is too short to allow the trochanter to be fixed straight in superior location.

The capsule is then easily and widely exposed. In its anterior part, the fibers of the iliopsoas muscle are gently separated, and in its posterior part, the short external tendons are also separated from the capsule and preserved by a retractor.

The capsule is resected in two flaps. First, the posterior flap is removed which is facilitated by the positioning of the femur in internal rotation. Then, moving the femur in external rotation, the anterior flap is resected from the joint line to the intertrochanteric line. The hip can be dislocated by femoral adduction and external rotation across the table, the knee in flexion in order to minimize traction on the sciatic nerve. The proximal femur is elevated by a retractor put under the posterior aspect of the trochanter, and the femoral neck is cut according to the preoperative

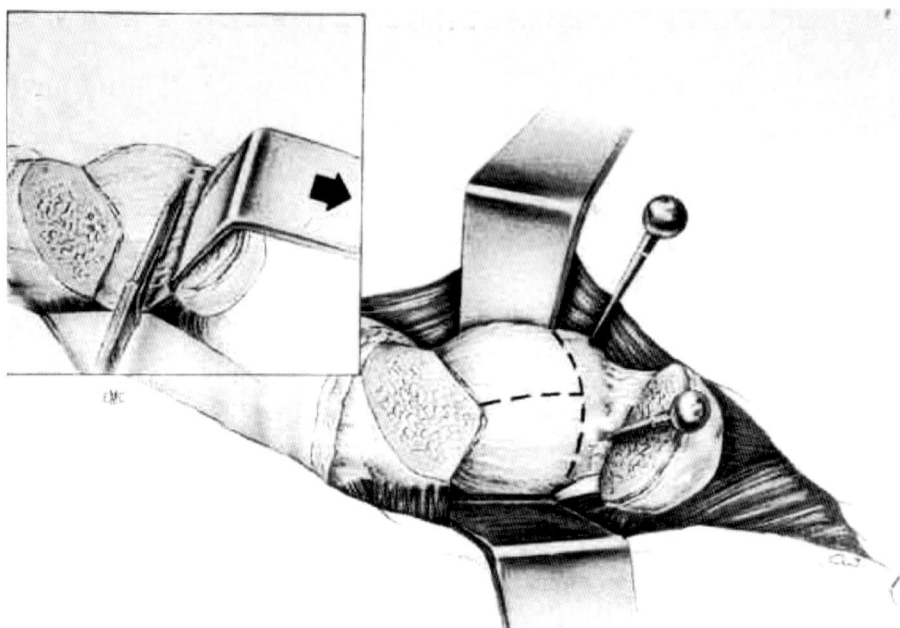

Fig. 7.2 The capsule is separated from the gluteus medius and the trochanter elevated superiorly
and posteriorly

planning. The exposure of the acetabulum is improved by the repositioning of the
pins if need be and by the use of a hook retractor inserted under the inferior margin
of the acetabulum after the resection of the transverse ligament. Preparation of the
acetabulum and of the femoral diaphysis are then made.

Reattachment of the Trochanter

To have a rigid fixation, stainless steel wires 12, or 14 gauge in strong and heavy
patient, are used. These wires must be elongated by at least 50 % under tension to
allow a balanced tensioning of the different wires.

Before implanting the femoral component, a drill hole is made in the femoral
cortex at least 2 cm below the trochanter section to allow the distal advancement of
the trochanteric fragment if desired. Three vertical stainless steel wires are run
through this hole into the medullary canal and go out through the femoral neck,
one anterior two posterior. The wires are properly arranged in the femoral canal and
stabilized in the medial part of the femoral neck by putting them in two small
notches made in the anterior and posterior cortices. After the implantation of the
femoral component, a transverse wire is passed around the femoral neck or under
the lesser trochanter.

After reduction of the hip, the trochanteric fragment is pulled down with a grasp
to appreciate its positioning (Fig. 7.3). If the trochanter can be pulled distally to its

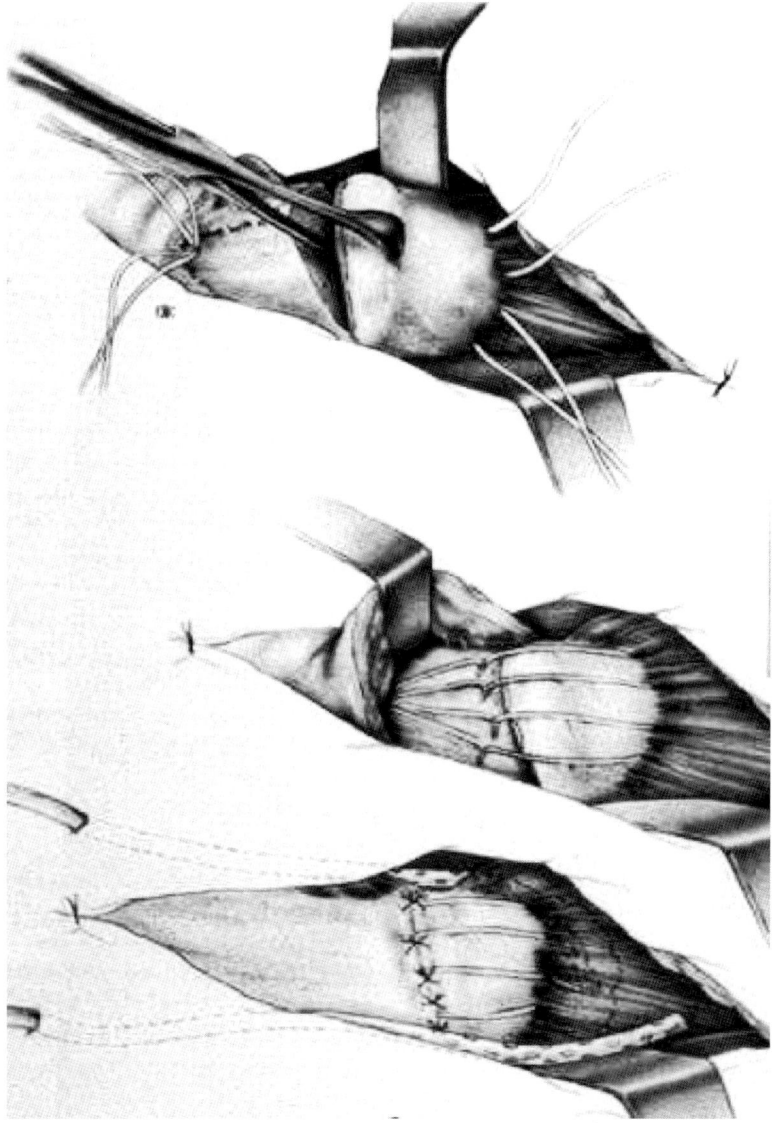

Fig. 7.3 The trochanter is pulled down and the abductor muscles tension is assessed. The metallic wires are passed over the trochanter and distributed on its surface. At last, they are tightened with an equal tension

original situation, that means that it is necessary to advance it distally and vertically to restore a proper tension to the gluteus medius and to increase its level arm. In this case, using an oscillating saw, a small triangular resection of bone is made on the lateral cortex of the femur. Then the vertical wires are passed over the trochanter through the abductor tendon very close to the bone. They are fixed to their distal end below the trochanteric section using a Danis tightener. It is important to give each wire a strong and equal tension to make sure that the trochanter is strongly applied on its bed. The last transversal wire is passed around the trochanter under the anterior part of the gluteus medius and tightened. The wire twists are cut short, applied on the bone under the tubercle of the vastus lateralis, and covered by the suture of the muscle tendon. The twist of the transversal wire is also bended and impacted into the lateral cortex of the trochanter to avoid any impingement with the soft tissues.

Advantages of the Transtrochanteric Approach

In every case, the transtrochanteric approach to the hip offers broad simultaneous exposure of the femur and acetabulum. This exposure allows for safe, precise, and consistent orientation of the components and perfect resection of the osteophytes all around the bony acetabulum to avoid impingement. Also, this approach allows for preserving integrity of periarticular muscles and specially the short external rotator muscles that are the main actors to prevent posterior dislocation of the artificial hip. All of these advantages act together to minimize the risk of postoperative dislocation because of the muscular integrity and balance and because of the proper positioning of the components. That explains why even using a 22 mm femoral head our personal dislocation rate is very low: 0.1 % in primary arthroplasty and 1.5 % in revision. It is also important to notice that transtrochanteric approach helps the surgeon to improve the geometrical reconstruction of the artificial hip allowing an acute restoration of the center of rotation, the leg length, and the level arm of the abductor muscles.

In difficult primary total hip arthroplasties, transtrochanteric approach demonstrates all its advantages facilitating dislocation, exposure, and muscle balancing in patients with ankylosis or fusion, protrusio acetabuli, proximal femoral deformities and specially coxa vara deformity, severe developmental dysplasia, or abductor muscle laxity. In severe proximal femoral deformities (Figs. 7.4 and 7.5), it is possible to go back to a normal anatomy through the remodeling of the metaphysic allowed by the trochanteric osteotomy.In revision procedures, trochanteric osteotomy facilitates hip dislocation, resection ofsoft tissue contracture and scarring that interfere with exposure, and removal of existing components and cement. As well, it also facilitates the insertion of the new components, particularly when extensive reconstruction of both acetabulum and femur is needed.

But in revision arthroplasty, the contact between the trochanteric fragment and its bed may be very narrow and cancellous bone absent or of poor quality. In this case, bone union will be very late and a stronger fixation by adding a trochanteric claw plate to the wiring will be safer (Fig. 7.6). We also use this trochanteric claw plate for the treatment of ununited trochanter [7]. As well, it is also better to graft the bone bed with autograft if available or allograft.

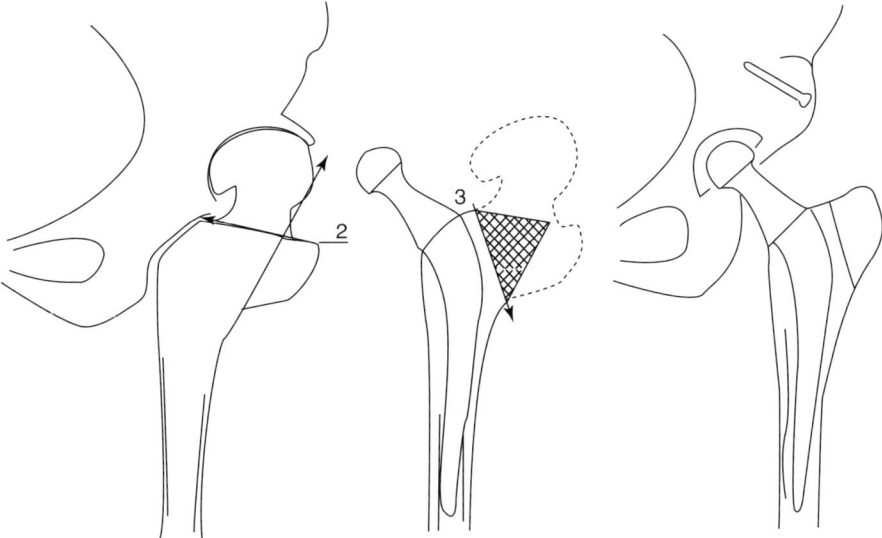

Fig. 7.4 Proximal femur remodeling during total hip replacement after proximal femoral osteotomy performed previously

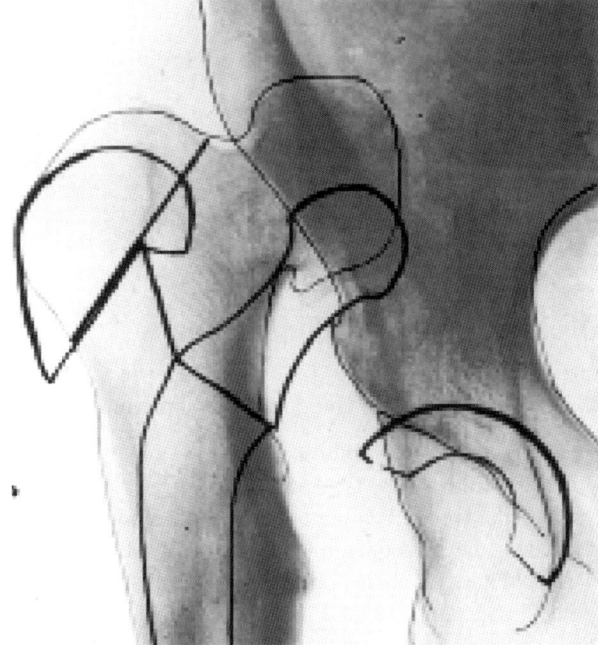

Fig. 7.5 Proximal femur remodeling during total hip replacement for Crowe type 4 dislocation

Fig. 7.6 In this case of femoral revision with a double sheath technique, the trochanter has been reattached with wires and a trochanteric claw plate to get a more resistant and more rigid fixation

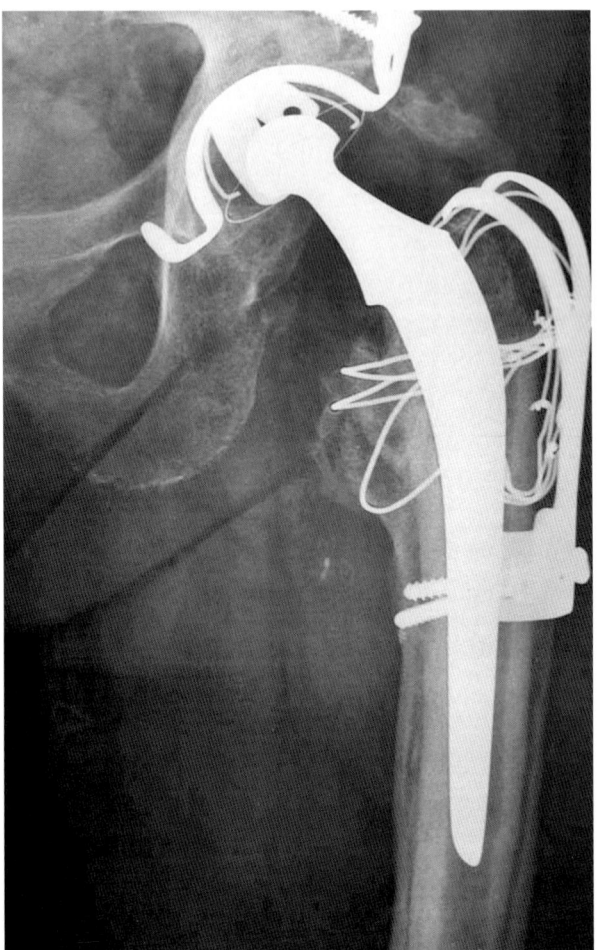

Disadvantages and Complications

Only three are specific and due to the approach itself:

- The bleeding is slightly increased.
- The operative time is 15 min longer.
- A partial weight bearing for 6 weeks is absolutely necessary until the trochanter is healed; the surgeon must be guided by the radiographic appearance. The patient should not start abduction exercises against gravity until the radiographs confirm that the trochanter has united. The patient can then begin to use one crutch for walking.

The other disadvantages are usually due to technical errors; poor surgical technique, generally in cutting or reattaching the trochanter; and using weak or brittle wires. A suitable wire may be of stainless steel 1.2 or 1.4 in section with a great plasticity (the range of elongation to failure in conventional tensile test must be about 100 %).

The trochanter approach is a relatively difficult technique requiring a long training, but if meticulously done, complications such as trochanteric pain, bursitis, and nonunion of the trochanter are rather scarce.

Bursitis practically never occurs when the wire twists are cut short and hidden under the muscles. The rate of nonunion can be as low as 0.1 % in primary arthroplasty and 1 % in revision for an experimented surgeon (personal data). In a series of total hip replacement performed by senior as well as young surgeons, the nonunion rate was 3 % [8].

Contrary to what J. Charnley [1] used to say, the trochanter cannot unite within 3 weeks without imposing restriction. Six weeks are necessary to get bone union, and full weight bearing must be delayed at a minimum of 6 weeks in primary surgery and frequently more in revision.

Discussion

Three issues must be debated there. Are there still some indications for transtrochanteric approach in 2013? What kind of osteotomy is the best? What is the safest trochanter reattachment technique?

In our experience, transtrochanteric approach still is the safest and the most efficient approach to implant properly the components while restoring in any case the hip architecture. Despite these evidences, this approach has progressively been abandoned all over the world and it is interesting to understand why. The major reason was a high rate of nonunion reported in some publications [9]. In our experience, nonunion was always due to a poor technical realization or a nonrespect by the patient of the partial weight bearing period. Actually, these two causes can be easily avoided by an attentive learning of the surgical technique and by a good information delivered to the patient. The other main reason is that nowadays total hip replacement is presented as a simple surgical act and that patient wants to have a rapid recovery. So, most of primary total hip arthroplasties and many revisions are done without osteotomy of the greater trochanter. For the surgeon, the advantages of not doing a trochanteric osteotomy are many. The blood loss and operating time are usually less, nonunion is eliminated, and wires or cables are not needed. As the hip is a very compliant and forgiving joint, the short-term clinical results of THA performed without trochanter osteotomy are usually good even so either some muscles have been damaged or the joint architecture has not been properly restored. If the patient is able to walk and if pain is relieved, both the patient and the surgeon are happy. At the same time, we also see in the current debates around hip replacement that one of the major concerns of surgeons still is postoperative dislocation. Some of them are now trying to address this problem through some modifications of the implant design like dual mobility cup or larger femoral head. We can bet that using new implants, they will experiment new problems as always seen in the orthopedic experience since 40 years. We still are convinced that the best way to prevent dislocation remains to preserve all the muscle and to restore the hip architecture. According to these guidelines, we still use the transtrochanteric approach in each difficult case and routinely if the patient is able to respect partial weight bearing. Some authors [2] think that in selected cases involving difficult primary or revision procedures, osteotomy of the greater trochanter has distinct advantages, and in a few situations, it is mandatory. According to this, they use only in few and difficult cases this approach and as they do not practice this technique routinely, they have much more complications. That is the reason why we recommend to surgeons who want to learn this technique to start with simple cases and always with the good tools to cut and repair the trochanter.

Second issue is to define the best kind of osteotomy. In fact, partial osteotomy of the trochanter, either anterior or posterior, is only transmuscular approach and must be excluded from this discussion. The exposure is less large and it is impossible to modify the muscular location or tension. Regarding true transtrochanteric approach, the choice has to be made between plane and biplane osteotomy [3, 10]. Biplane osteotomy theoretically offers a better stabilization of the trochanter when reattached and a wider bone contact surface to facilitate the fusion. But the biplane osteotomy has for us more drawbacks than advantages. First, it does not allow for adjustment of trochanter location, and second, there is a risk of fracture of the trochanter at the summit level. For these reasons, we always perform a plane osteotomy.

Last issue is the choice of the safest technique for trochanter reattachment. Many techniques and tools have been used. It is important to understand that the greater trochanter is a weak bone submitted to important muscular tension. The reattachment technique must resist to these traction forces, anteriorly and proximally, while preserving the great trochanter [6]. Several techniques have been described. Screws are not suitable in this application because of the weakness of the lateral cortex of the trochanter. The technique using only one wire seemed to be successful for Harris [11], but it is for us unsafe to use only one wire cables grip have demonstrated that they can be responsible for polyethylene wear [12] in case of breakage and further more are difficult to tighten. For us, stainless steel wire remains the best choice. We use usually three vertical wires and one transversal wire. These four wires can be distributed on the trochanter surface to face the traction force and they do not damage the trochanter.

As a conclusion and with the experience of all the other approaches, we can say that it is possible to perform a simple total hip replacement with a good result without a trochanteric osteotomy but a transtrochanteric approach will always allow for a better restoration of the hip architecture and will preserve all the muscles. In difficult cases, the transtrochanteric approach is always more efficient and safer. The only problem is to maintain the possibility for the young surgeon to be educated and trained with this approach to allow them to appreciate its huge advantages and consequently to avoid its drawbacks.

References

1. Charnley J (1972) The long-term results of low-friction arthroplasty of the hip performed as a primary intervention. J Bone Joint Surg Br 54:61–76
2. Archibeck MJ, Rosenberg AG, Berger RA, Silverton CD (2003) Trochanteric osteotomy and fixation during total hip arthroplasty. J Am Acad Orthop Surg 11:163–173
3. Courpied JP, Desportes G, Postel M (1991) A new trochanteric osteotomy method for a postero-lateral approach (330 operations with posterior transosseus and paramuscular curved approach). Rev Chir Orthop Reparatrice Appar Mot 77:506–512. French
4. McGrory BJ, Bal BS, Harris WH (1996) Trochanteric osteotomy for total hip arthroplasty: six variations and indications for their use. J Am Acad Orthop Surg 4:258–267
5. Hersh CK, Williams RP, Trick LW, Lanctot D, Athanasiou K (1996) Comparison of the mechanical performance of trochanteric fixation devices. Clin Orthop 329:317–325
6. Kerboull M (1994) Arthroplastie totale de hanche par voie transtochanterienne: Editions Techniques. Encyclopedie Medico-Chirurgicale, Techniques Chirurgicales-Orthopedie-Traumatologie. Elsevier, Paris
7. Hamadouche M, Zniber B, Dumaine V, Kerboull M, Courpied JP (2003) Reattachment of the ununited greater trochanter following total hip arthroplasty. The use of a trochanteric claw plate. J Bone Joint Surg Am 85:1330–1337
8. Kerboull L, Hamadouche M, Courpied JP, Kerboull M (2004) Long-term results of Charnley-Kerboull hip arthroplasty in patients younger than 50 years. Clin Orthop 418:112–118
9. Nercessian OA, Newton PM, Joshi RP, Sheikh B, Eftekhar NS (1996) Trochanteric osteotomy and wire fixation: a comparison of 2 techniques. Clin Orthop 333:208–216
10. Wroblewski BM, Shelley P (1985) Reattachment of the greater trochanter after hip replacement. J Bone Joint Surg Br 67:736–740
11. Jensen NF, Harris WH (1986) A system for trochanteric osteotomy and reattachment for total hip arthroplasty with a ninety-nine percent union rate. Clin Orthop 208:174–181
12. Hop JD, Callaghan JJ, Olejniczak JP, Pedersen DR, Brown TD, Johnston RC (1997) The Frank Stinchfield Award. Contribution of cable debris generation to accelerated polyethylene wear. Clin Orthop 344:20–32

Chapter 8
A Modified Anterolateral, Less Invasive Approach to the Hip: Surgical Technique and Preliminary Results of First 103 Cases

Herve Hourlier

Abstract One hundred and three (103) consecutive primary total hip arthroplasty cases were treated with a modified, anterolateral, minimally invasive approach and were prospectively followed to determine short-term outcome. A minimal dissection soft tissue-preserving technique was achieved by a slide osteotomy of the lateral facet of the greater trochanter through skin incisions which were less than or equal to 10 cm in length. The capsule was not excised but incised in the same line as the gluteus minimus. The prospective study group was operated in 2003 and compared to a retrospectively matched control group of patients, operated in 2002, that had received total hip arthroplasty using a conventional-sized lateral approach. The mini-incision, anterolateral, modified approach was found to be as safe as the standard approach while providing quicker patient recovery. The minimal invasive approach was not associated with improper component placement.

Keywords Total hip replacement • Anterolateral surgical exposurey • Postoperative bleeding

Introduction

Minimally invasive surgery (MIS) is thought to provide important benefits in comparison to traditional extensile exposure. Except for cosmetics, MIS is associated with lower blood loss, lesser pain, and faster rehabilitation. Because of the consistently reported high success rate of conventional total hip arthroplasty (THA), it is imperative to critically appraise these new MIS techniques. A variety of mini-incision techniques in THA currently exist. Besides an innovative, controversial, two-incision technique, assisted by fluoroscopy, and promoted by R. Berger [1],

H. Hourlier
Service d'Orthopédie, Polyclinique de la Thiérache,
Route de Féron, 59212 Wignehies, France
e-mail: h.hourlier@gmail.com

D.G. Poitout, H. Judet (eds.), *Mini-Invasive Surgery of the Hip*,
DOI 10.1007/978-2-287-79931-0_8, © Springer France 2014

various single-incision techniques via anterior, anterolateral, or posterior approaches have been described. The results which have been reported differ in relation to the type of approach. For instance, improper component position has been reported with the mini-incision, posterior approach [2]. So far, studies using the mini-incision anterior or anterolateral approach have not reported this adverse outcome [3, 4]. Although no significant positive influence on recovery from decreased incision length was observed for the anterolateral approach in a recent report [4], minimizing incision length specifically for such a surgical approach should theoretically decrease muscle damage and risk of injury to both the superior gluteal nerve and to the transversal branch of the circumflex artery, both of which are located at the limits of the incision. Damage to these elements has been associated with abductor muscle weakness, delayed recovery, and persistent limp [5, 6]. These adverse consequences should be theoretically reduced by a smaller incision that respects the safety zone for the nerve and causes less trauma to the muscles [5, 7].

This chapter describes my surgical technique and reports on the early postoperative results of the first consecutive 103 THAs performed with a modified, anterolateral, minimally invasive approach. Outcome is compared retrospectively to a matched patient cohort of 88 cases performed with the conventional lateral approach.

Materials and Methods

Patient Population

From a pool of 165 consecutive primary total hip arthroplasties, 103 consecutive hips (102 patients) were selected for the minimal incision THA technique, defined as a skin incision that was less than or equal to 10 cm in length. Excluded from this prospective study group were patients with previous surgery of the joint or those suffering from post-traumatic arthritis, rheumatoid arthritis, and postinfectious arthritis. The mini-incision group of 103 hips was operated between February 2003 and March 2004 and compared with a population of 88 hips (88 patients) that were operated in 2002 with the use of a conventional incision (15–20 cm) via a modified, anterolateral approach. The control group was retrospectively matched using the same inclusion criteria as for the study group. Baseline data is listed in Table 8.1. No statistical significant differences between the two study arms were found with respect to age, gender, body mass index, preoperative functional Postel and Merle d'Aubigné score (PMA score) [8], fraction of patients operated for primary osteoarthritis (OA), or preoperative hemoglobin level. While care was exerted in matching the patients, there were more ASA 3 patients in the control group than in the study group (Table 8.1). All arthroplasties were performed cementless with use of a tapered rectangular titanium stem (SL-Plus®, Plus Orthopedics Ltd., Rotkreuz, Switzerland) and a press-fit metal-backed acetabular component. The bearing surfaces were mainly alumina ceramic-on-ceramic in both groups. All surgeries were performed in the same laminar airflow theater by the same surgeon under general

Table 8.1 Baseline
characteristics in
the two groups

	Mini incision	Standard incision	
Baseline values	$N = 103$	$N = 88$	p-value
Gender (M/F)	49/54	50/38	0.205*
Age	67.0 ± 10.9	67.3 ± 12.6	0.838**
Primary OA (%)	85.4 %	78.4 %	0.928**
BMI (kg/m²)	27.2 ± 4.1	27.9 ± 4.4	0.272**
Preop PMA score	10.0 ± 1.4	9.6 ± 1.6	0.206***

*Chi-square, **Mann-Whitney, ***Fisher exact

anesthesia and using a hemocare device. The same rehabilitation protocol was prescribed. Immediate full weight bearing was allowed. All patients were free to ambulate the second day after the surgery. The use of one crutch was prescribed for minimum 1 month. The follow-up program included a clinical and x-ray exam done after 6–12 weeks and at 1 year. The PMA score was used to establish the postoperative rating. No patients in either group were lost to follow-up.

Statistical Analysis

Data were evaluated with Statistica 6.1 (StatSoft Inc., Tulsa, OK, USA). Alpha was chosen at 0.05. Between-group comparisons were performed with the Student's t-test or the Mann-Whitney test for continuous variables, the Mann-Whitney test for ordinary scaled variables, and the chi-square and Fisher exact test for nominal scaled variables.

Surgical Technique

Patient Positioning

The patient is placed on the operating table in the lateral decubitus position with the pelvis locked perpendicular to the table. The entire leg and hip are prepared and draped. A supplementary sterile pouch is dressed in front of the operating table in order to place the leg in a vertical position at the femoral preparation step.

Incision

The skin incision is made longitudinally in a straight line over the greater trochanter from 3 cm above the tip to 5 cm below (Fig. 8.1). The fascia lata is divided in a straight line and the gluteus maximus is splitted in line upwards. This division is

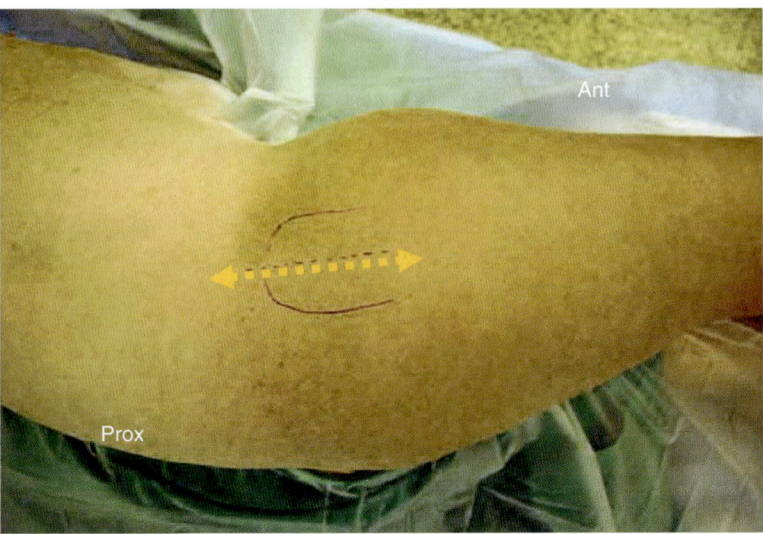

Fig. 8.1 Skin incision

extended 3 cm proximal and distal beyond the limits of the skin incision; the incision of the trochanteric bursa reveals the anterior and posterior borders of the great trochanter and its attaches. Using cutting diathermy, a longitudinal incision is made to divide the tendinous periosteum over the great trochanter centered midway between the anterior and posterior margins and extended distally in the middle of vastus lateralis tendon to a point 1 cm beyond the vastus ridge. The incision extends proximally to divide, in an anterior curved direction, 1/3 anterior of the gluteus medius muscle in direction of the fibers and not more than 2 cm above the tip of the great trochanter (Fig. 8.2).

Approach

With use of an oscillating saw, an osteotomy of the lateral aspect of the great trochanter is performed in an upward direction from the vastus ridge in order to preserve the transverse branch of the lateral circumflex artery (Fig. 8.3). The trochanteric fragment is vertical, linear, about 5–8 mm thick and carries with it the continuation of the anterior part of the gluteus medius and the vastus lateralis. It is attached proximally to the anterior part of the gluteus medius and distally to the anterior half of the vastus lateralis. Rotating the extremity laterally achieves a medial slide of the fragment which is then mobilized anteriorly to expose the gluteus minimus and the capsule which are incised in the same line. The distal part of the gluteus minimus is detached jointly from the capsule and from its femur insertion. The proximal part of the incision is extended along the femoral neck in an anterior direction toward the

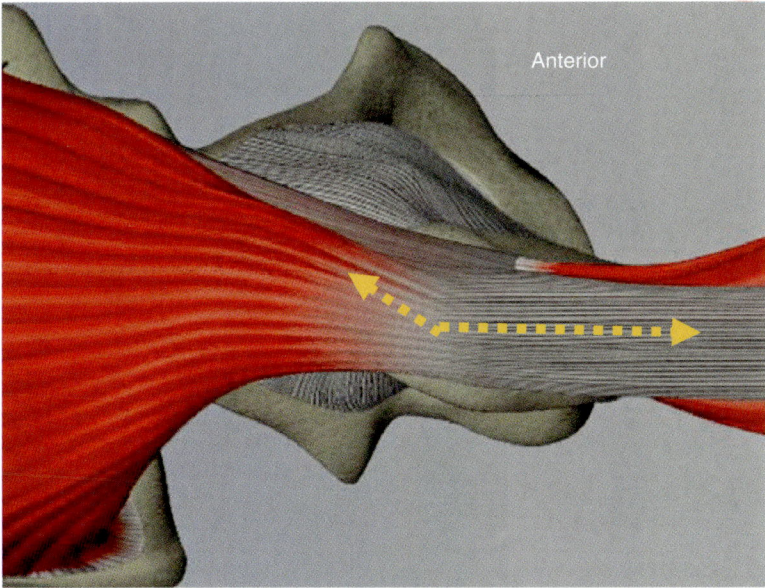

Fig. 8.2 1/3 gluteus medius-1/2 vastus lateralis digastric anterior flap developed with bony intermediate junction created by osteotomy of the lateral facet of the greater trochanter

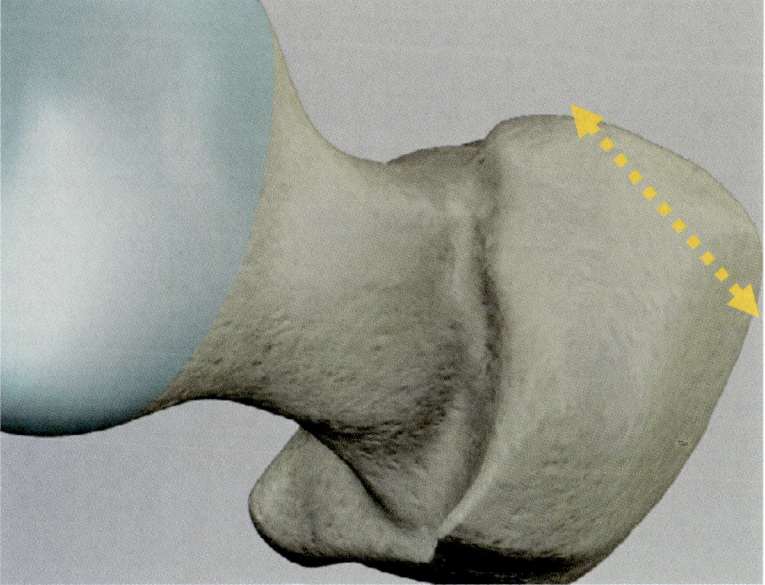

Fig. 8.3 Osteotomy of the lateral facet of the greater trochanter

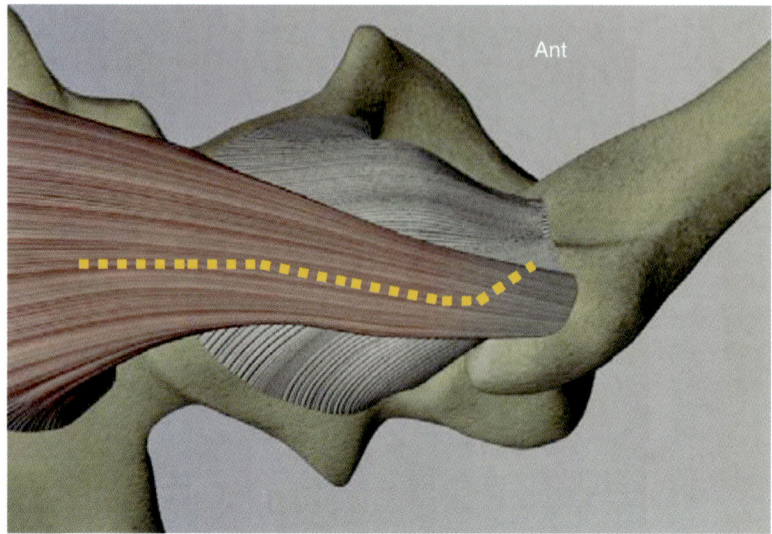

Fig. 8.4 Split of the gluteus minimus and incision of the capsule in the same line

superior acetabular rim (Figs. 8.4 and 8.5). The femoral neck is transected in situ or after dislocation; then, the femoral head is excised.

Acetabular Exposure

After removal of the femoral head, the position of the leg is adjusted to give the exposure of the acetabulum. In most cases, lateral rotation and slight flexion of the hip give the best access. After excision of the labrum, two spiked Hohmann retractors are inserted over the anterior and posterior edges of the acetabulum (at 4 and 8 o'clock). Then the capsule can be released if necessary to the medial border of the femur. A Steinman pin or a self-retaining retractor is placed proximally to retract the capsule and the gluteus muscles (Fig. 8.6). The entire acetabular cavity can now be seen and remnants of the labrum are excised.

The acetabular bony preparation is performed with an angled reamer handle designed for use in minimally invasive surgery of the hip. Either a curved impactor through the incision directly or a straight impactor through a separate percutaneous incision is used to insert the cup in proper position.

Femoral Exposure

The femoral preparation is made with the foot placed vertically. The exposure is provided by two spiked Hohmann retractors, one placed on the medial and the

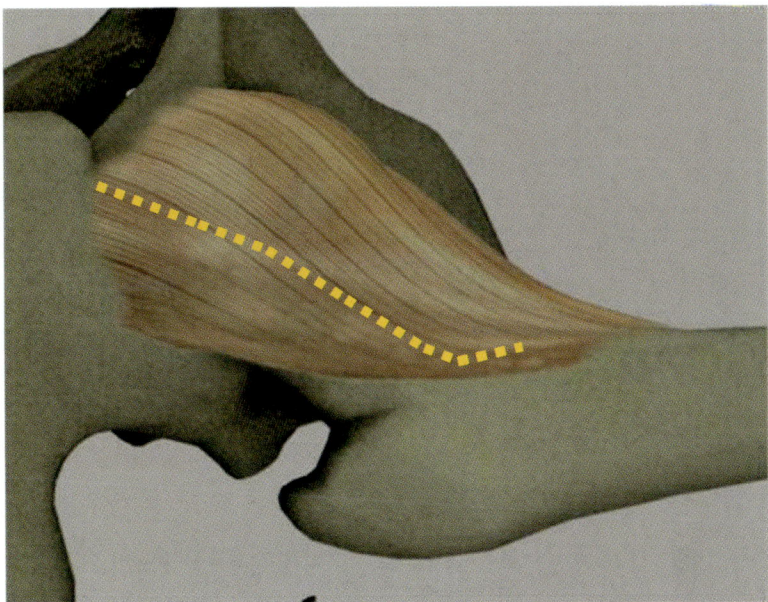

Fig. 8.5 Line drawing of the capsule incision

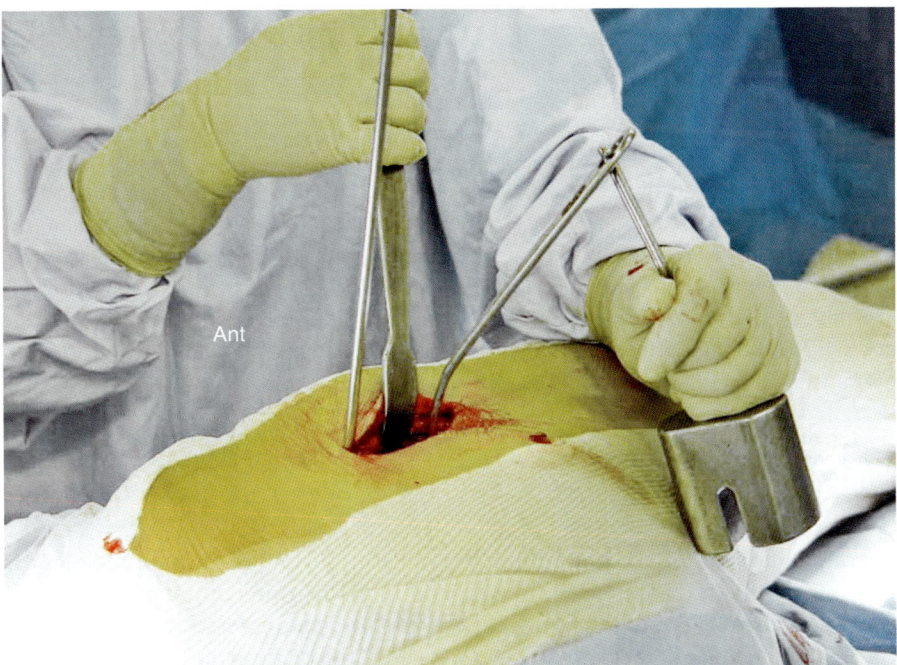

Fig. 8.6 Acetabular exposure is provided by two spiked Hohmann retractors and a Steinman pin

Fig. 8.7 Operative aspect
before the closure (right hip)

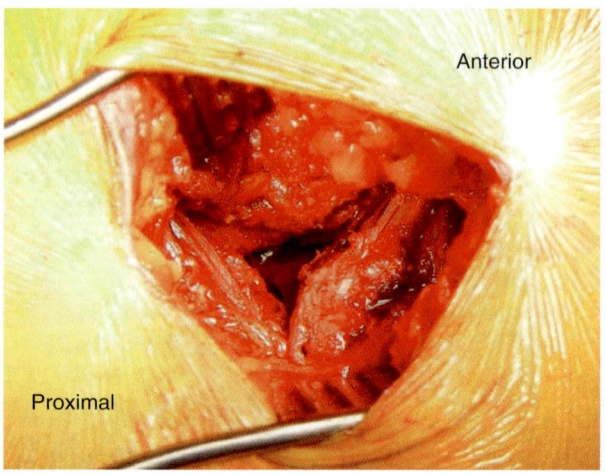

other posterolateral side of the femur. A third spiked Hohmann can be placed
advantageously under the posterior femoral neck anterior to the ventral gluteus
medius part to prevent muscle damage possibly encountered by the femoral rasps.
Sharp-cutting femoral rasps of rectangular cross section and increasing size are
used with a pneumatic hammer to achieve direct anchorage by press fit. After satisfactory trial reduction with a trial device the definitive prosthesis is inserted and
the hip is reduced.

Closure

The closure is made in layers. The capsule and the gluteus minimus are jointly
sutured and can be reattached to the femoral bone (Fig. 8.7). Then the trochanteric
slide fragment is reattached to the proximal femur by a single cerclage wire
(monofilament 1.2 mm steel) passed anteriorly to the stem of the prosthesis through
drill holes. The twist of the metal knot is placed under the vastus ridge to prevent
trochanteric bursitis related to the cerclage wire (Fig. 8.8). The fascia lata, gluteus
fascia, subcutaneous tissues, and skin are closed in usual fashion.

Clinical Results

Average time for surgery was 62 min for study group and 63 min for the control
group ($p = 0.51$). No decreased time related to the learning curve was observed
between mid-practice in the mini-incision group. Postoperative day 1 after surgery, the hemoglobin level was 11.8 g/l for the study group and 11.6 g/l for the

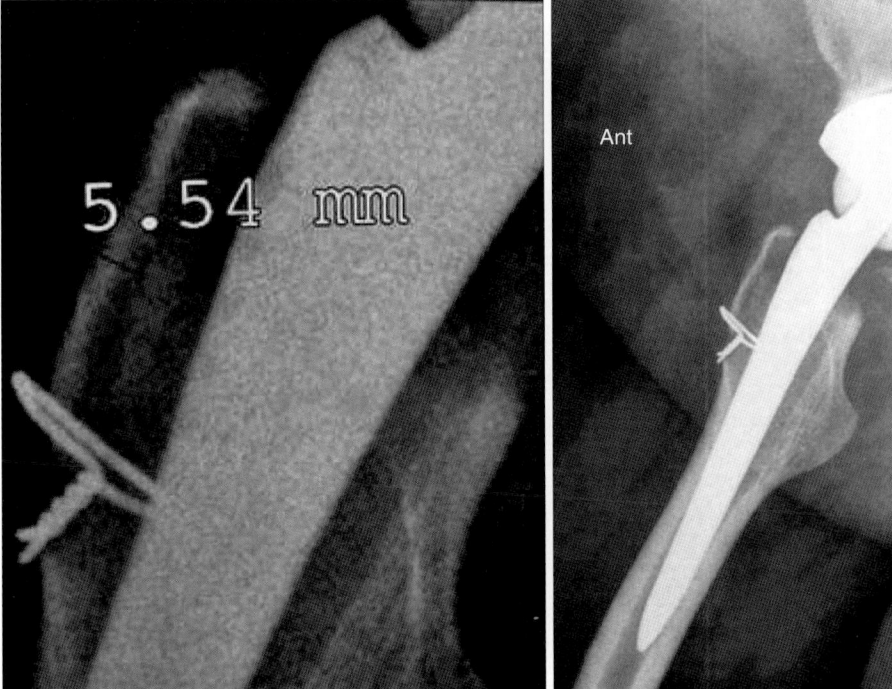

Fig. 8.8 The lateral radiograph and focus show the reattachment of the trochanteric fragment with a wire

control group ($p = 0.42$). However, fewer patients in the study group received blood autotransfusion with hemocare (16 % vs. 49 %, $p < 0.001$), and the amount of blood transfused was less for the study group (119 ml vs. 130 ml, $p < 0.001$).

Three patients were transfused with allogenic blood in the MIS group; all were older than 80 years. One of these patients had a preoperative hemoglobin level at 10 g/l; the two others received transfusion just prior to discharge (Table 8.2).

Complications

In the both groups, no wound healing, nerve palsy, infection, femoral fracture, or prosthetic dislocation complications emerged. In the mini-incision group, one mal-positioned ceramic inlay required revision after 6 days. The inlay was replaced successfully. In each group, two cases of deep vein phlebitis were detected just prior to discharge.

Table 8.2 Comparison of hemoglobin levels and rates of blood transfusion in the two groups

Blood loss	MIS N = 103	Standard incision N = 88	p-value
Haemoglobine level			
Preoperative (gr/l)	14.2 ± 1.3	13.8 ±1.1	.074
Postoperative day-1 (gr/l)	11.8 ±1.4	11.6 ±1.5	.423
Drop level	16.9 %	15.9 %	
Hemocare device			
% Patients re-infused with hemocare	16.5	46.6	.000
Average volume of re-infusion (ml)	117 ± 32	130 ± 78	
No. of patients having receiving allogenous blood transfusion	3	6	.313

Table 8.3 Comparison of operating time and outcomes in the two groups

Result	Mini incision group N=103	Standard incision group N=88	p-value
Surgical time (min)	61.9±14.5	62.7±12.9	.508*
Length of hospital stay (days)	8.3±3.5	9.6±3.6	.000*
Patients discharged home (%)	78.4	60.2	.01**
PMA at 1 year	17.3±.9	17.1±.8	.423*

Values are given as mean±SD
*Mann-Whitney, **Chi-square

Clinical Evaluation

Hospitalization time was 8.3 postoperative days for the study group and 9.6 postoperative days for the control group ($p<0.001$). One year postoperatively, the PMA score was 17.3 for the study group and 17.1 for the control group ($p=0.42$) (Table 8.3).

Radiographic Results

Component position was not different between the two groups. Immediate postoperative X-rays showed excellent overall alignment and fit of all the components in the mini-incision group. The femoral stems were in neutral alignment in 95 cases and in varus alignment of less than 5° in the remaining eight cases. Cup abduction angle averaged 38.5° with all components between 30° and 48°.

At the last follow-up, no component in either group has shown migration.

Discussion

The direct lateral approach is attractive for THA since it provides excellent visualization of both acetabular and femoral regions through a comparatively small skin incision [9]. The quality of component placement is afforded by the straightforward and direct line of sight characteristic of the operative procedure. The risk of dislocation is lower than with posterior approach [6, 7, 9]. The trans-gluteal approach, with splitting of 1/3 of the abductors, was originally introduced by Bauer [10] to prevent muscle damage encountered when performing THA via the traditional Watson Jones, anterolateral intermuscular approach, between the gluteus medius and the tensor fascia lata.

Intraoperative damage to the anterior abductors and difficulties inherent in effectively repairing muscle to the bone have long been associated with the Watson Jones approach. In addition, the risk of postoperative heterotopic bone formation has been linked to this approach, despite it does not necessarily affect clinical outcome [7]. The direct lateral approach for THR was popularized by Hardinge [11], despite the inconvenience of delayed recovery and clinical abductor weakness. Postoperative abductor insufficiency after abductor split has been ascribed to injury to the vascular and nerve supply to the muscles [5, 7], when the safety zone of the superior gluteal nerve is not respected and muscle damage is incurred by dehiscence of the reattachment suture line [12]. The amount of the disruption in the abductors, which is related to the surgical point of entry into the abductor muscle mass, has been also considered as crucial [13].

For these reasons, several modified direct lateral approaches, including various flap designs and suture repair methods, have been proposed. To maintain the flap continuity and reinforce the tendinous junction between the gluteus medius and the vastus, McFarland and Osborne [14] originally advised attachment of some spikes of the bone to the trochanteric periosteum tendon [13]. In a similar way, McLauchlan [9], followed by Dall [15], has proposed greater trochanteric osteotomies with reattachment of bone to bone. However, the device of fixation for reattaching the fragment to the bone can cause potential trochanteric bursitis which may need reoperation. For instance, in using the Dall approach, Learmonth [16] reported a rate of 11 % of reoperation to remove the cerclage wire.

One distinct advantage of the partial anterior trochanteric osteotomy proposed by Ganz is that it preserves the whole gluteus medius and allows a rapid recovery of the abductor power. The nonunion of the fragment can occur but without any functional effect [17].

The minimally invasive approach described in this chapter is different from the other anterolateral exposures in several ways:

- The dissection is minimal.
- Approach to the hip is no vascular.
- Soft tissues connections between the fascia lata and gluteus medius and between the gluteus minimus and capsule are preserved.

- Each and every one of the gluteus muscle (maximus, medius, and minimus) is split in the direction of their fibers. Only the distal part of the insert of the gluteus minimus is detached from the femur.
- The capsular tissue is not excised but incised in the same line as the gluteus minimus is. Thus, at the time of the closure, it can be sutured jointly with the gluteus minimus and reattached back to the femur through osseous sutures.

Sliding of the lateral facet of the greater trochanter gives a number of advantages:

- This surgical approach is technically easy to perform.
- Dissection is minimized with all the soft tissue attachments conserved between the fascia lata and the gluteus medius. The use of thermal cautery to peel off the internal rotators from the greater trochanter is reduced. The internal rotators can be released with preservation of their attachments to the trochanteric fragment.
- Splitting and elevating the gluteus medius-vastus lateralis anterior flap avoid stretching damage to the glutei and/or the tensor fascia muscles.
- The junction of the flap is positively reinforced, especially in the face of a thin gluteal-vastus aponeurosis covering the greater trochanter. Hence, the continuity of the flap can be maintained with the strength of reattachment to the femur possibly increased.
- The risk of vascular injury of the transversal branch of the lateral circumflex artery is decreased. Moreover, the blood supply of the greater trochanter is preserved and the risk of nonunion of the fragment possibly reduced [6].
- The greater trochanter is in full view for femoral rasping and stem insertion. The point of entry into the femur is exposed in direct line of sight and then can be easily unlocked. Through a such approach, the penetration of the wing part of the SL-Plus® stem into the trochanter is not a concern because the partial trochanteric slide osteotomy facilitates the entrance and allows to achieve repeatedly a regular position of the stem in the longitudinal axis of the femur.
- The reattachment of the fragment, when closing, allows regulation for the tension of the internal rotators maintained to the fragment. In our department, a single cerclage wire has been used in over 400 total hip replacements. Several failures of union occurred with no evident functional repercussion. Therefore, no reattachment was required. Conversely, some breakages of the cerclage wire were associated to adverse repercussions needing a reoperation. For this reason, nonabsorbable osseous stitches are now preferred (Ethibon 6).

The learning curve for the modified direct lateral minimally invasive approach is by no means demanding; the technique is not much different than a standard total hip. Neither a specific operating table nor an unusual setting for the surgeon is required. Except for the curved acetabular reamer, conventional instruments are used. Any stem design can be implanted through this approach, but the Zweymüller stem offers the advantage that the stem fixation is unrelated to the level of the femoral neck osteotomy. Moreover, the Woodpecker pneumatic hip broaching system facilitates femoral preparation, sizing, and good primary fixation of the stem.

The hospital stay and the speed of functional recovery in this current report are far from the spectacular results described by Berger with the innovative two-incision technique, but the cohort of patients is different and the rehabilitation protocol has not been altered for this comparative study. Importantly, however, this mini-incision, anterolateral approach was not associated with any increase in the number or type of complications compared to the historic matched control group. Most reports of MIS surgery include an increased incidence of femoral fractures, component mal-position, and early reoperation rates. Additionally, the mini-incision lateral approach offered a faster recovery to patients (1 day less in hospital) while reducing the total medical costs since 78.9 % of the patients were discharged directly to home in the mini-incision group versus 60.2 % of the patients in the standard group.

The mini-modified anterolateral approach is applicable to most patients, as dem-onstrated by our ability to use the approach in 62 % (103/165) of consecutive pri-mary hip operations in this commencing series. For obese patients, the skin incision can easily be extended by 2 cm in each direction to make the exposure easier.

Conclusion

The mini-incision, anterolateral modified approach was found to be as safe as the standard approach while also achieving a shorter length of stay in hospital and a higher rate of discharge to home. We did use neither intraoperative fluoroscopy nor computer guidance, yet the quality of component positioning was not compro-mised. Sliding of the lateral facet of the greater trochanter minimizes dissection and facilitates implantation of a tapered stem in proper position. By combining a customized small incision size, a careful component positioning, as the use of hard-bearing surfaces demands it, and the famous, fully proven Zweymüller stem, we anticipate long durability of the arthroplasty, in addition to the advances in the early postoperative outcomes that we have documented in this study, compared to our prior surgical approach.

Perspective

This study has initiated at our institution a radical change of perioperative blood management in total joint arthroplasty. Because our results provided no evidence supporting the usefulness of perioperative cell saver system, we decided to stop the use of reinfusion system during primary THR in 2005.

At that moment, any autologous blood transfusion was implemented in our unit as preoperative autologous blood donation was not utilized either.

We replaced autotransfusion systems by a chemoprophylaxis in selected patients to reduce blood losses and transfusion requirements.

This blood-sparing transfusion strategy allowed us to perform a consecutive series of 221 unilateral less invasive THAs without any blood transfusion [18].

Thereafter, we also abandoned the use of wound drain because the volume collected by suction drain was regularly little.

Acknowledgments   The author thanks Peter Fennema for statistical analysis and contribution.

References

1. Berger RA (2003) Total hip arthroplasty using the minimally invasive two-incision approach. Clin Orthop 419:232–241
2. Woolson ST, Mow CS, Syquia JF, Lannin JV, Schurman DJ (2004) Comparison of primary total hip replacements performed with a standard incision or a mini-incision. J Bone Joint Surg Am 86:1353–1358
3. Kennon RE, Keggi JM, Wetmore RS, Zatorski LE, Huo MH, Keggi KJ (2003) Total hip arthroplasty through a minimally invasive anterior surgical approach. J Bone Joint Surg Am 85(Suppl 4):39–48
4. Mahoney O, Asmaya I, Kinsey T (2004) The effect of incision size on clinical outcomes and recovery after total hip arthroplasty with the antero-lateral approach. AAOS, San Francisco
5. Duparc F, Thomine J, Dujardin F, Durand C, Lukasiewicz M, Muller J (2003) Hemimyotomie antérieure – anatomie chirurgicale et technique. Ann Ortho Ouest 35:46–49
6. Ritter MA, Harty LD, Keating ME, Faris PM, Meding JB (2001) A clinical comparison of the anterolateral and posterolateral approaches to the hip. Clin Orthop 385:95–99
7. Mulliken BD, Rorabeck CH, Bourne RB, Nayak N (1998) A modified direct lateral approach in total hip arthroplasty: a comprehensive review. J Arthroplasty 13:939–949
8. Merle D'Aubigné R (1970) Cotation chiffrée de la fonction de la hanche. Rev Chir Orthop 56:481–486
9. McLauchlan J (1984) The stracathro approach to the hip. J Bone Joint Surg Br 66:30–31
10. Bauer R, Kerschbaumer F, Poisel S, Oberthaler W (1979) The transgluteal approach to the hip joint. Arch Orthop Trauma Surg 95:47–49
11. Hardinge K (1982) The direct lateral approach to the hip. J Bone Joint Surg Br 64:18–19
12. Swenson O, Sköld S, Blomgren G (1990) Integrity of the gluteus medius after the transgluteal approach in THR. J Arthroplasty 5:57–60
13. Frndak PA, Mallory TH, Lombardi AV (1993) Translateral surgical approach to the hip: the abductor muscle "spilt". Clin Orthop 295:135–141
14. McFarland B, Osborne G (1954) Approach to the hip: a suggested improvement on the Kocher's method. J Bone Joint Surg Br 36:364–369
15. Dall D (1986) Exposure of the hip by anterior osteotomy of the greater trochanter. A modified anterolateral approach. J Bone Joint Surg Br 68:382–386
16. Learmonth ID, Allen PE (1996) The omega lateral approach to the hip. J Bone Joint Surg Br 78:559–561
17. Nezry N, Jeanrot C, Vinh TS, Ganz R, Tomeno B, Anract P (2003) Partial anterior trochanteric osteotomy in total hip arthroplasty: surgical technique and preliminary results of 129 cases. J Arthroplasty 18:333–339
18. Hourlier H Fennema P Line B (2008) A new blood -saving plan for less invasive primary total hip replacement. Orthopaedics 31

Chapter 9
Minimally Invasive Posterior Approach: Technical Evaluation, Initial Results and Follow-Up at Two Years

Stephan Procyk

Abstract Posterior approach of the hip is commonly used in English-speaking countries. Although it provides an excellent exposure of the joint and functional results, this technique is often criticised for its high related rate of prosthetic dislocation especially when using smaller 22.2 femoral head. The technical optimisation designated by "minimally invasive access" preserves its advantages without compromising the clinical and radiological results. The prospective clinical series presented in this chapter gives evidence to the benefits of posterior minimally invasive access, with a significant improvement of the outcomes in terms of pain and functional recovery and a reliable and reproducible prosthetic implantation. Continuous visual control of each gesture reduces the rate of perioperative complications, incompatible with routine use, and minimal tissular aggression allows to obtain the results expected from a minimally invasive technique at short and long term.

Keywords Lateral decubitus • Posterior access of the hip • Piriformis • Minimally invasive surgery of the hip • Posterior tendinous-capsular flap

Introduction

The posterior approach [1], frequently used in English-speaking countries since the 1950s, is commonly utilised because it is a technique that is easy to learn and reproducible. It offers an excellent exposure of the hip joint and constitutes a safe and easy access even in difficult cases (important stiffness, protrusions). It allows total prosthesis fitting without significant tissular damage, provided trochanterotomy is performed.

S. Procyk
Department of Orthopaedic Surgery, Clinique du Ter, BP71,
Ploemeur Cedex 56275, France
e-mail: stefprocyk@aol.com

D.G. Poitout, H. Judet (eds.), *Mini-Invasive Surgery of the Hip*,
DOI 10.1007/978-2-287-79931-0_9, © Springer France 2014

Various types of incision have been described, based on *Langenbeck's* princeps access [2] used in 1874 for the drainage of a sceptic hip arthritis.

When optimised [3], this approach allows minimally invasive surgery with opening the gluteus maximus following the axis of its fibres, minimal aggression of pelvi-trochanteric muscles and their reconstruction using a tendinous-capsular flap.

As shown by the presented series, this technique rules out the main disadvantage of the posterior access that of its associated high rate of dislocation and permits easy implantation of larger (32, 36, 40) head diameter.

Material and Method

The author initiated this experiment of less aggressive surgery in 1998. Since emphasis has been put on the respective advantages of numerous techniques, it was interesting to objectively demonstrate the posterior access ones.

Patient Selection

One hundred consecutive cases were performed during the period since from May 2005 to February 2006, there were no exclusion criteria. One implant was used: press-fit cup and a straight, tapered cementless titanium stem with two offsets (standard and lateralised).

Surgical Technique

Preoperative Schedule

A preoperative schedule is made for each patient using the tracing; it allows an estimation of the implant size, correction of potential length inequality and restoration of the femoral offset (one of the key points to prevent dislocations).

Position of the Patient

The operating table is maintained strictly horizontal. The patient is lying in lateral decubitus and held firmly; the pelvis is fixed vertically using a reference bar positioned perpendicular to the table axis, so as to align the superior anterograde iliac pins. This position helps to obtain the triaxial benchmark and facilitates the determination of appropriate implant orientation [4]. In such a lateral decubitus

Fig. 9.1 The piriformis tendon and gluteus medius reclined by the Hohmann

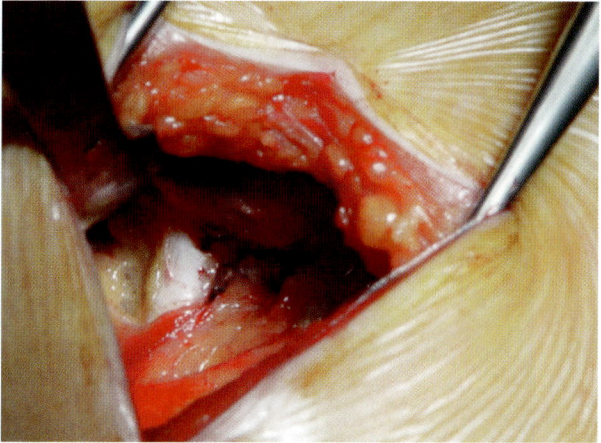

position, the pelvis is fixed in flexion by the holding devices [5]. It must be kept in mind to obtain appropriate acetabular anteversion (essentially in male patients).

After sterilisation of the area, the relative difference of length is made after knee palpation.

Incision

Positioning the incision is essential for optimal reduction of the incision size and, at the same time, ensures adequate visualisation, minimal aggression and correct implant position. With the hip and the knee slightly bent, the femoral axis is drawn and the top of the greater trochanter is marked after palpation. The posterior edge of the gluteus medius is palpated through the skin; this location is optimal for the incision, constituting an *angle of 20° with the femoral axis* (Fig. 9.1); this technique has been previously described by Swanson [5]. The incision length is calculated as the third of the patient's body mass index (BMI). An outline tracing with a window may be utilised for marking facilitation [6].

Surgical Access

A straight incision is performed along the previously determined line; the final length depends on the amount of fat and the compliance of the tissues; the subcutaneous tissue is cut perpendicularly with particular care to avoid detachments and to control haemostasis. The gluteal fascia is incised following the axis of gluteus maximus fibres (Fig. 9.2). The gluteus maximus muscle is bluntly splitted in the direction of its fibres, beginning from its femoral part where the muscle is

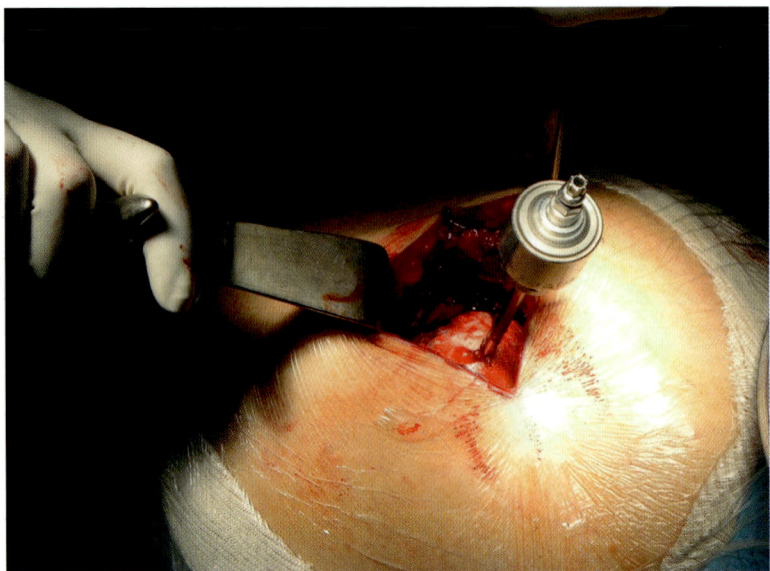

Fig. 9.2 Head removal

thin; the fascia lata must be always preserved. An autostatic retractor is carefully placed. The short internal rotators are hidden by an adipose layer but the fig may be easily palpated, just beneath the gluteus medius (Fig. 9.3). The fat layer is cut along a line that goes *along the piriformis up to the femur* and then shows a slight posterior *curve* (Fig. 9.4).

A Hohmann retractor is placed under the gluteus medius. The piriformis is stretched by an internal rotation of the hip until it is adequately tensed, and then it is detached at the place of its femoral insertion in the piriformis fossa (if it appears retracted) or preserved. The posterior capsular joint is then opened following the axis of the piriformis tendon, after the femoral insertion (Fig. 9.5). External rotators (superior gemelli and even the internal obturator) are detached from their insertion but must remain adherent to the capsular flap; the inferior gemelli and the quadratus femoris are preserved. If the hip is not too stiff, this may be sufficient to allow femoral dislocation (flexion, adduction, internal rotation) while preserving the median circumflex pedicle. A threaded pin (external fixator) is drilled in the femoral head for future atraumatic extraction after section of the femoral neck, so as to avoid the placement of cumbersome instruments inside the incision. At this stage, the dislocation remains difficult due to the tension of the capsular reinforcement ligament (which protects the inferior gemelli and quadratus femoris, hence the median circumflex vascular pedicle that circulates in the quadratus femoris); its femoral insertion, clearly visualised, is cut, liberating the femur.

This step-by-step muscular disinsertion helps to preserve a maximum of muscles.

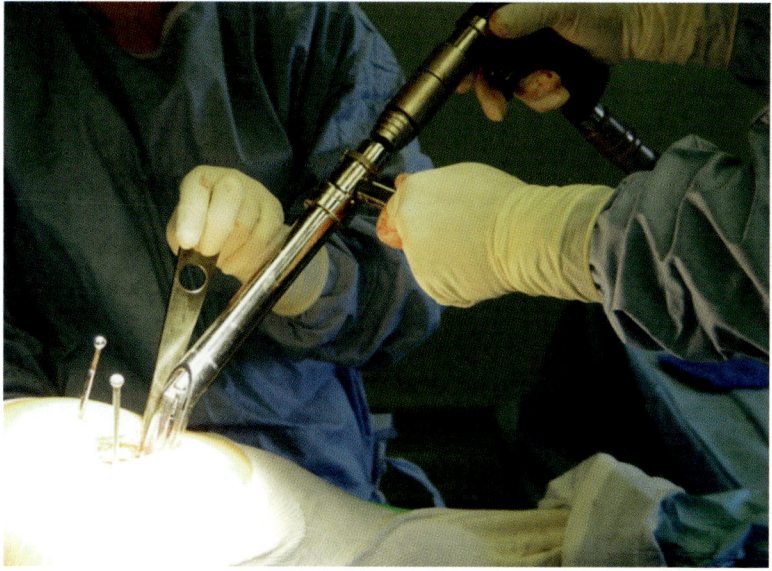

Fig. 9.3   Some necessary tools for acetabular preparation

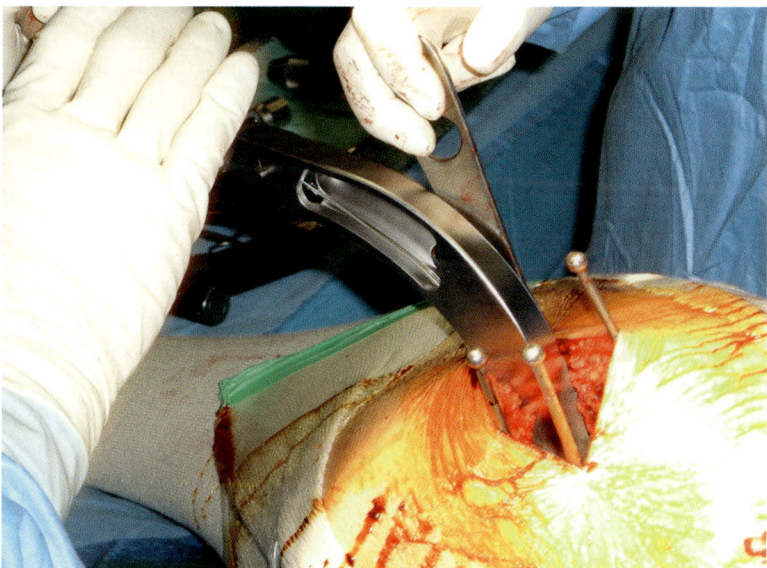

Fig. 9.4   Acetabular implantation

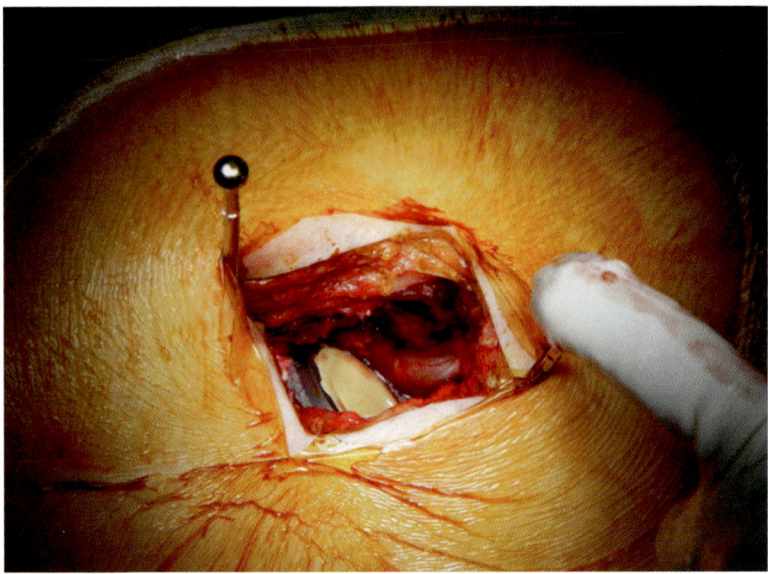

Fig. 9.5 Final view of the implant

Femoral Neck Sectioning, Acetabular Exposure

The femoral neck osteotomy is performed in accordance with the preoperative schedule, using a minimum of retractors in order to reduce tissular tensions.

After extraction of the femoral head, the autostatic retractor is taking-off; the acetabulum is exposed by *posterior* reclination of the tendinous-capsular flap which is maintained by two pins. The first is placed in the posterior inferior iliac spine and the second is placed *higher* in the posterior spine, the sciatic nerve being protected by this flap. To achieve the exposure, another pin is placed above the acetabulum in order to move the superior capsula and suprajacent muscles apart. Acetabular labrum, osteophytes, pathologic tissues or a thickened capsular joint are excised. A Hohmann retractor is placed above the anterior spine and maintains anterior femoral dislocation [7]. The acetabulum is exposed; its bottom is cleaned from the pulvinar and osteophytes; finally, the acetabular transverse ligament is systematically excised.

Drilling

The drilling may begin lightly, in a centred manner, so as to obtain a hemispheric cavity. The use of a staggered drill support helps this action in accordance with the necessary orientation without tension or rubbing in the distal part of the wound and cancels the risk of mechanical burning of the skin. The last drilling gives visual information on the acetabular covering and the tactile sensation helps to tell on the quality of the bone, which gives an estimation of the primary stability of the implant.

Acetabular Implantation

When the cavity reaches the bleeding subchondral bone, the acetabular component is implanted using a curve impactor that prevents orientation errors (it does not press on the wound edges or on the femur). With the posterior access, the posterior part of the cupula is introduced first by a *sliding* movement. By helicoid rotation, it is placed into the acetabulum by a *sliding* of potentially interposing soft tissues. The correct position of the cupula is based on the external benchmarks constituted by the orthogonal lines of the operating room and the orientation stems fixed on the impactor; these are useful when setting the inclination and the anteversion of the component. At this stage, impinging osteophytes are excised, which definitively liberates the joint. Then, the definitive insert (admitting the larger diameter head) is installed and impacted using a staggered tool.

Femoral Preparation

In order to expose the proximal extremity of the femur, it must be positioned in compliance with the incision axis: the knee is bent at 90° and the tibia is vertical. This position is the reference for the stem orientation. A lip retractor is placed under the neck and a small Hohmann retractor is inserted under the gluteus, so as to clear the site of instrumental penetration at the trochanteric level. Classical femoral preparation is carried out: the femoral duct is opened by a dedicated box chisel, starting the perforation into the greater trochanter to avoid varisation of the stem, followed by successive rasping with the smallest rasp indicating the working axis, and also introduced into the greater trochanter. When the final rasp is correctly seated, tests are performed using testing components with different neck lengths and offsets, and the access permits easily the use of larger head diameter; the stability and the length of the limb are estimated by another knee palpation (*starting reference*). All retractors are removed in order to facilitate testing and liberate soft tissues. Once testing components are removed and sizes are selected, the definitive components are implanted on the same basic principle of retraction and *tissue preservation*.

Suture/Closure

After achievement of the femoral reduction (if the hip anatomy is restored), the posterior capsular flap with its adherent tendons spontaneously takes its initial anatomic position. Capsula, piriformis tendon and superior gemellus are fixed up and ahead, using several absorbable sutures passing under the greater trochanter and through the gluteus medius tendon. The whole apparatus is covered by the repositioned adipose flap. We recommend the use of an intra-/extra-articular suction drainage. Then, absorbable suture is performed on the gluteus maximus, the fascia and the subcutaneous tissues. The skin is coapted by an intradermic continuous suture that prevents secondary problems of clip or stitch ablation and allows the use of hyaluronic acid dressings that accelerate healing.

Postoperative Management

The primary goals are, for patients, no pain and regain their healthware quickly, a rapid recovery program with a preoperative education achive those [8]. Pain may easily be controlled by IV perfusions that combine Prodafalgan and ketoprofen during 24–48 h and then by oral stage II analgesic agents. Drainage is stopped after 48 h. The preoperative education about physical therapy accelerates the patient's recovery [9]. A complete standing posture the next day and passive and active rehabilitation start immediately. The patient's autonomy is not restrained and the hospital stay duration is limited to strict security requirements and recovery of sufficient autonomy for returning home.

Results

- The operation time is into standards (48 ± 9 min); the intraoperative blood loss is 175 ± 82 ml, the bearing surfaces utilised are ceramic head (28 diameter) on polyethylene in 24.3 % and ceramic on ceramic in 75.7 % (BIOLOX forte 32 diameter), and the procedure is a real limited incision: length of skin incision is 7.8 ± 1.6 cm.
- No perioperative event such as bone lesion and neurological or vascular damage has been observed in this series.
- No significant clinical complication occurred such as dislocation, hematoma (no need to surgery) or sepsis. Only a localised bleeding at the drain site was reported. No difference in lower limb length (no correction) has been observed.

Intraoperative	Acetabular fracture (1)
Early postoperative (general)	Anaemia transfusion (1), anaemia infusion (1), gastric bleeding anaemia (1), transfusion (1)
Early postoperative (local)	Haematoma (2), local bleeding (2), superficial bleeding/ ecchymoses (2)
1 week ($N=100$)	Local bleeding (1)
3 months ($N=99$)	Haematoma (1)
	Pain (1)
	No information (1)
2 years ($N=91$)	Fracture (1, injury)
	Stem revision (1, haematogenic sepsis)

- Radiological results: The leg length difference is optimised. No verticalisation of the acetabulum potentially induced by the minimised access has been observed or acetabular abduction >50°. Satisfactory anteversion was obtained; all components were located between 15° and 30°. In this series, femoral stems were adequately oriented (zero varus or valgus) in 72 %; osteo-integration was perfectly achieved with all components; no edging was visible after 1 year, indicating an absence of ossification.

Leg length difference		
None	78	(77.2 %)
Ipsilateral longer	19	(18.8 %)
Ipsilateral shorter	4	(4.0) %
Leg length difference		
Ipsilateral longer	4.7 ± 2.8 mm	(2–15 mm)
Ipsilateral shorter	5.8 ± 3.0 mm	(3–10 mm)

CUP position (°)	% of patients ($N = 100$)
40–50	98
<40	2
>50	0
Stem position (°)	% of patients ($N = 100$)
Neutral	72
Varus up to 5	28
Varus up over 5	0
Valgus up to 5	0
Valgus up to over 5	0
Stem (2 years) FUP	No signs/some abnormalities
Radiolucent lines	
Osteolysis	81/19
Atrophy	99/1
Hypertrophy	82/18

- Functional results: The evolution was rapid owing to the use of stage II analgesic drugs at D2–D3. Analgesics were spontaneously stopped between D12 and D20. Ninety-five percent of the patients were walking with a walking stick at D5; they get up from sitting on a chair without any help at D6 and started walking upstairs at D6. Joint liberation resulted in rapid recovery of mobility and articular amplitude—80 % of the final result as soon as D6. At D20 (between D10 and D30), stable monopodal pressure is achieved. Patients spontaneously returned to sedentary activities at D15 and mild work at D30 and regained their health quickly. Younger patients returned to occupational activity between D40 and D60.

Harris Hip Score

	Preoperative	3 months	2 years
Function	21 ± 7	44 ± 5	46 ± 3
Total score	37 ± 10	96 ± 6	98 ± 7

mean ± SD points, max. 100 points

Overall ROM

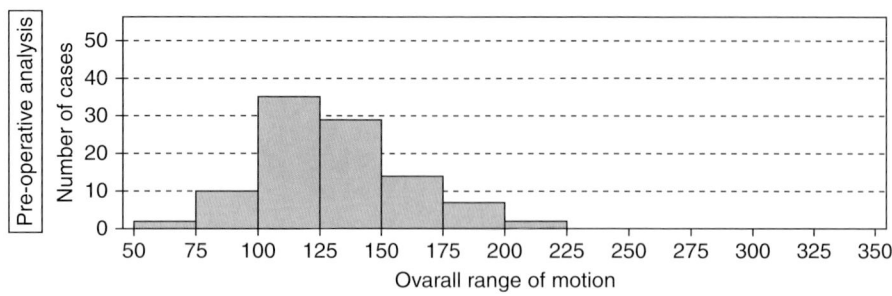

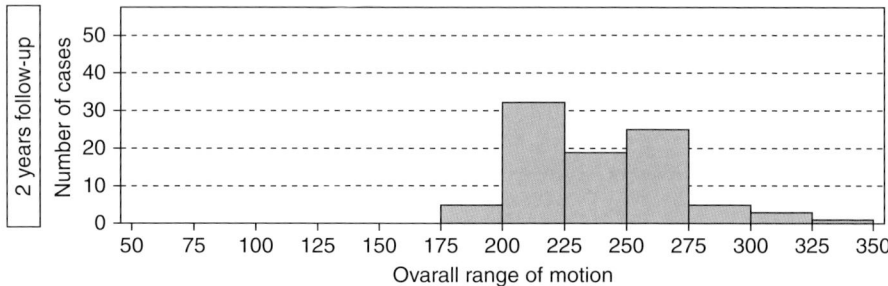

WOMAC

	Preoperative	3 months	2 years
Pain	45±18	89±14	99±7
Stiffness	36±19	80±19	98±8
Physical activity	35±17	85±13	97±9
Total score	37±16	86±13	97±8

Discussion

A first studied series [10] necessitated a longtime implementation because the radiological criterion of morphologic appropriateness of the implant imposed a very strict selection based on metaphyseal anatomy (a straight stem with metaphyseal filling was utilised, and two offsets might be selected). This stem implying lower cut of the femoral neck, it necessitated too important pelvi-trochanteric disinsertion hence a posterior access that should be considered an optimised reduced posterior access rather than a real minimal-posterior access. In this prospective series at 2 years follow-up, the results show significantly improved early outcomes, maintained in time and surgical reliability: no major postoperative event or secondary complication was reported. Nevertheless, to avoid catastrophic complications [11], the training duration is long, both for the surgeon and his assistants; the operative

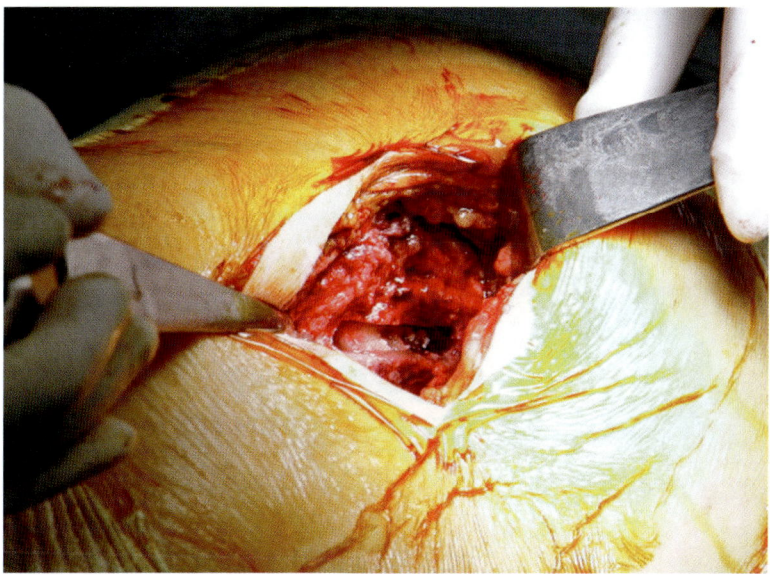

Fig. 9.6 Expose the femur, less retractors, straightway

time is prolonged by 15 min with each gesture being more difficult; the procedure lasts 1 h on average. Implantation is reliable and reproducible.

Demystifying the surgical procedure but with a confident relationship to the patient (as proved by the use of the WOMAC), this technique means a reduction in the duration of hospital stay; it implies an easy postoperative management and the patients' rapid return to their usual activities, with optimal comfort and with time an improved result in terms of health-related quality of life.

Conclusion

The mini-posterior access is recommended by the author since it results in an excellent cure of the acetabulum and allows working in the femoral axis, even in difficult cases (stiffness, protrusion, obese or muscular patients). The visual control of each gesture is always possible. In case of perioperative complication, widening the access is always easy, without any additive damage.

The current utilisation of Zweymüller-type straight implants participates in a progression towards true posterior mini-access and more preservation for the pelvi-trochanteric muscles (Figs. 9.6 and 9.7). The strictly rectilinear femoral stem with a four-angled section and reduced anteroposterior dimensions allows working in the femoral axis; its use is highly versatile, nonlimited by the femoral geometry; its upper position allows reducing the femoral neck section and minimising the external rotators disinsertion.

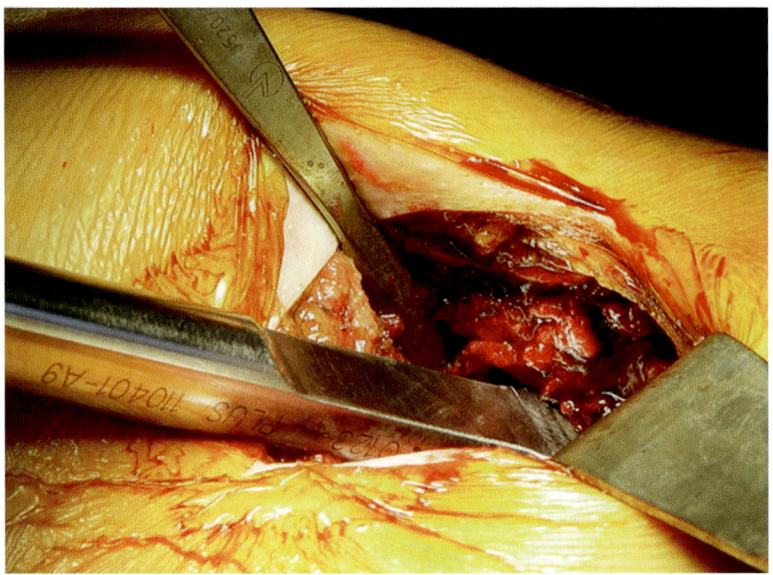

Fig. 9.7 Broaching the femoral shaft

The results are comparable to published data; the mini-posterior approach does not in any way compromise the good short-term performance of the Zweymüller-type implants [12, 13].

Among the panel of multiple approaches described today or under experiment, this is a less hazardous access that really reduces postoperative pain, accelerates functional recovery and minimises tissue aggression. In terms of cosmetics, it is noteworthy that the scar is located on a part of the body that is invisible for the patient and hidden by clothes. The psychological benefit is important and the patient's compliance in terms of rehabilitation is rapidly obtained. From the patient's point of view, minimisation of pain and care demystifies this surgery and maximises the feeling of confidence and comfort.

All in all, this approach is easy, predictable, and can be planned, giving way to comfort.

References

1. Harris WH (1975) A new approach to total hip replacement without osteotomy of the greater trochanter. Clin Orthop Relat Res 106:19–26
2. von Langenbek B (1874) Veber die Schussverletzungen des Huttgelenks. Arch Klin Chir 16:263
3. Berry DJ, Berger RA, Callaghan JJ, Dorr LD, Duwelius PJ, Hartzband MA, Lieberman JR, Mears DC (2003) Minimally invasive total hip arthroplasty. Development, early results and critical analysis. J Bone Joint Surg Am 85A:2235–2246

4. Stillwell WT (1987) The posterior approach. In: Stillwell WH (ed) The art of total hip arthroplasty. Gruwe ad Strattou Inc, Orlando, pp 217–256
5. Swanson TU, Hanna RS (2003) Advantages of cementless THA using minimally invasive surgical technique. Presented at the 70th annual meeting of the AAOS, New Orleans, Felmang
6. Bush JL, Thomas PV (2007) Limited incision posterior approach for total hip arthroplasty, AAOS monograph series 36. pp 47–55
7. Hartzband MA (2006) Posterolateral minimal incision for total hip replacement. MIS techniques in orthopedics. Springer, New York
8. Dorr DL (2006) The new process of total hip replacement. Hip arthroplasty: minimally invasive techniques and computer navigation. Saunders Elsevier, Philadelphia
9. Crowe J, Henderson J (2003) Pre-arthroplasty rehabilitation is effective in reducing hospital stay. Can J Occup Ther 70:88–96
10. Procyk S (2006) Minimally invasive posterior approach. Technical evaluation and results. Interact Surg 1:35–40. Springer
11. Fehring T, Mason J (2005) Catastrophic complications of minimally invasive hip surgery. J Bone Joint Surg Am 87A:711–714
12. Zweymüller K, Schwarzinger UM, Steindl MS (2006) Radiolucent lines and osteolysis along tapered straight cementless titanium hip stems. Acta Orthop 77(6):871–876
13. Garcia-Cimbrelo E, Cruz-Pardos A, Madero R, Ortega-Andreu M (2003) Total hip arthroplasty with use of the cementless Zweylmuller Alloclassic system. J Bone Joint Surg Am 85A:296–303

Chapter 10
Hip Resurfacing and Anterior Approach

Philippe Piriou, Thierry Judet, Michel Serrault, and M. Mullins

Abstract In young and active patients, hip arthritis remains a challenge, whatever the improvements in materials, design, bone fixation and interfaces of total hip prosthesis (THR). Resurfacing provides a solution to at least some of these problems.

The anterior approach is the traditional approach for hip replacement in our department, as described and practised by Robert and Jean Judet since 1947, initially for the historical acrylic cephalic prosthesis and subsequently for all types of THR. It can be used as a truly minimally invasive approach as described by Siguier. This approach is now our standard approach for THR, allowing implantation without tendon or muscular section and taking advantage of the anteversion of both the neck and acetabulum.

This short prospective series involving just two types of implant does not allow any conclusion to be made about resurfacing concept: We have a favourable initial impression but as yet no answers regarding uncemented fixation, the prevention of bone trabecular modification, the incidence of metal ion release and so on.

On the other hand, the anterior approach performed on an efficient orthopaedic table seems to be recommendable. The only absolute contraindications are resurfacing combined with femoral osteotomy or cases where simultaneous metalwork removal is required.

So, for the marriage of resurfacing and a minimally invasive anterior approach, we have only great hopes for the implant but a complete and unrestricted faith in the approach!

Keywords Hip resurfacing • Anterior approach • Young patients, Robert and Jean Judet approach • Siguier minimal invasive approach • No tendon or muscles section

P. Piriou • T. Judet (✉) • M. Serrault • M. Mullins
Department of Trauma, Hôpital Raymond Poincaré,
Garches, Paris, France

D.G. Poitout, H. Judet (eds.), *Mini-Invasive Surgery of the Hip*,
DOI 10.1007/978-2-287-79931-0_10, © Springer France 2014

Introduction

What Are the Reasons for an Interest in Hip Resurfacing?

In young and active patients, hip arthritis remains a challenge, whatever the improvements in materials, design, bone fixation and interfaces of total hip prosthesis (THR). Resurfacing provides a solution to at least some of these problems; femoral neck elasticity and mechanical properties are preserved and the large head prevents dislocation. Moreover, it leaves the diaphyseal canal entirely intact to allow a more efficient and simple conversion to conventional total hip arthroplasty in the case of failure. Improvement of metal-on-metal bearings (McMinn [1–4], Wagner, Amstutz, etc.) since 1991 led us to suggest resurfacing for younger patients.

What Are the Reasons for the Anterior Approach?

It is the traditional approach for hip replacement in our department, as described and practised by Robert and Jean Judet since 1947, initially for the historical acrylic cephalic prosthesis and subsequently for all types of THR. It is basically a Hueter approach [3] which can be enlarged distally or, more frequently, proximally, as described by Smith-Petersen. On the other hand, it can be used as a truly minimally invasive approach as described by Siguier [4]. This approach is now our standard approach for THR, allowing implantation without tendon or muscular section and taking advantage of the anteversion of both the neck and acetabulum.

Since 2002, we have combined the accepted wide possibilities of anterior approach with the potential advantages of hip resurfacing [2].

Specificities and Details of Anterior Approach for Hip Resurfacing

The key point is to have a perfect view and instrumental control of both the acetabulum and femur for correct positioning and implantation.

Anatomic Basis

The anterior approach reaches the hip where the joint is the most superficial. It passes between two territories of innervation: the femoral nerve medially (sartorius (Sa), rectus femoris (RF) and iliopsoas (IP)) and the superior gluteal nerve laterally (tensor fascia latae (TFL), gluteus minimus (Gmin) and gluteus medius (Gmed)).

Neither muscle nor tendon is cut, except occasionally a release of the reflected tendon of rectus femoris. The anterior circumflex artery is the only vascular obstacle and is ligated.

Patient Set-Up and Operative Field Preparation

As always for the anterior approach, the patient lays supine on a fracture table which allows for any positioning of the lower limbs, particularly hyperextension, unlimited external rotation and adduction (Judet-Tasserit table, Collemier, France) (Fig. 10.1). Both antero-superior iliac spines and the pubis are accessible to palpation through the drapes, in order to confirm pelvic orientation. Likewise, palpation of the patella indicates the degree of external rotation. A rectangular 15×10 cm operative field is prepared, centred distally and laterally to the antero-superior iliac spine.

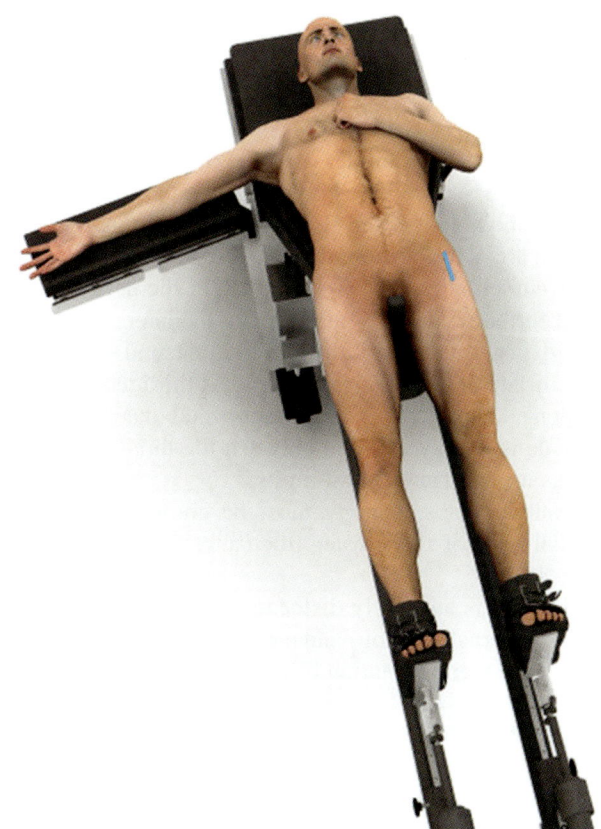

Fig. 10.1

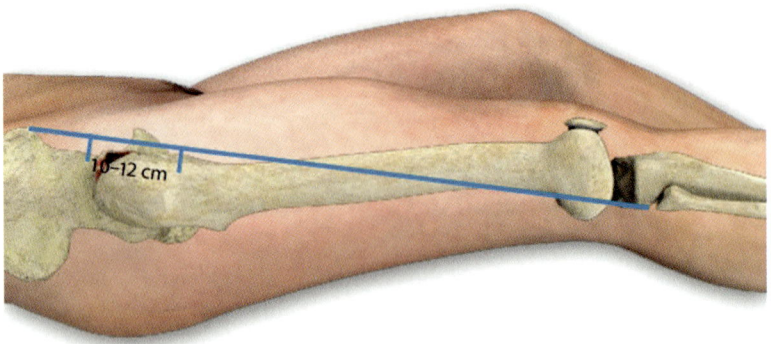

Fig. 10.2

Surgical Approach

A 10–12 cm oblique cutaneous incision is performed (Fig. 10.2). It begins one inch lateral to the anterior superior iliac spine and goes distally and slightly laterally along the anterior border of the TFL, and the aponeurosis is opened, leading to the muscle belly which is retracted laterally.

Anterior and posterior sheets of the RF are successively opened along the muscle lateral border.

The anterior circumflex artery is dissected out and ligated. The anterior hip capsule is then revealed; it is protected by an avascular fat pad which will be resected. On the medial side, the IP sheet is longitudinally opened, and the muscle and its tendon are elevated from the capsule with a periosteal elevator.

A curved retractor is inserted under the neck and, for improved comfort, somewhat further under the teardrop. On the lateral side, the periosteal elevator is introduced just under the Gmin, and a second curved retractor is placed over the supero-lateral aspect of the capsule. A third retractor is gently inserted under the RF tendon and applied on the anterior acetabular wall and the pelvic brim. The anterior capsule is widely exposed between the three retractors. The vastus lateralis origin marks its distal and lateral limits.

Anterior capsulectomy must be complete, particularly at the junction of the medial wall of the greater trochanter with the supero-lateral aspect of the neck (Fig. 10.3).

The hip is anteriorly dislocated by a combined effect of the table (traction and gentle external rotation) and a direct lever effect on the femoral head.

A 90° external rotation of the limb gives an access to the posterior aspect of the capsula (Fig. 10.4). A posterior circumferential capsulotomy is performed at mid-distance between the acetabular posterior margin and the inter-trochanteric posterior line.

This release allows a comfortable exposure of head and neck: The table maintains a position of 20° hyperextension, 90° or slightly more external rotation and a

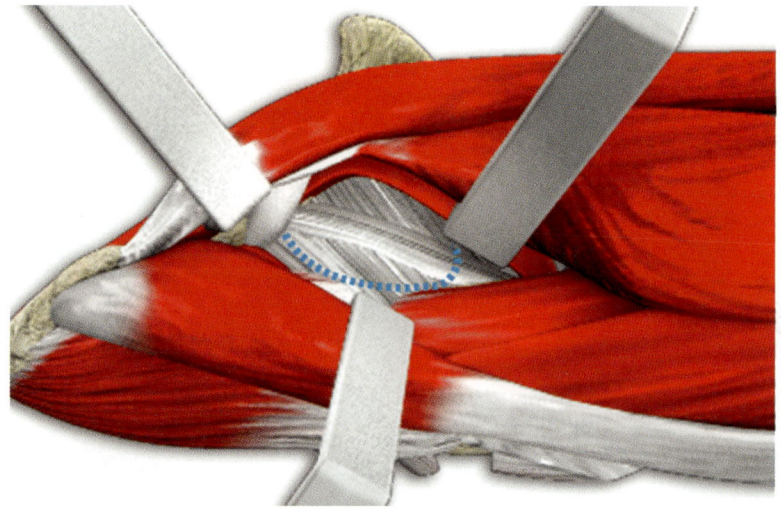

Fig. 10.3

degree of adduction ("femur position"). A strong double-curved retractor is applied behind the posterior inter-trochanteric line and a sharp retractor over the top of the greater trochanter to retract posteriorly the gluteus muscles and elevate the femoral metaphysis from the incision.

Complete peripheral control of the femoral head and neck facilitates the positioning and adjustment of the reaming axis. Next, the initial preparation of the femoral head is carried out.

Acetabular exposure: The hyperextension is corrected, and the leg is positioned horizontally with moderate external rotation to release the IP tension. The acetabulum is then exposed by a posterior displacement of the femoral metaphysis obtained by the lever effect of a strong double-curved retractor applied on the posterior wall and posterior column.

Standard reaming and implantation of the acetabular component are performed. The direct palpation through the drapes of the pelvic landmarks, pubis and the two antero-superior iliac spines allows a precise setting in both coronal and sagittal axes.

Femoral implantation: Definitive reaming and femoral implantation are performed in the "femur position". We have always cemented the femoral component, including the stem.

Reduction is obtained by gentle manipulation of the table, realignment of the leg, traction and internal rotation.

The wound closure on a suction drainage involves only the TFL aponeurosis, the subcutaneous tissue and the skin. Care must be taken to avoid accidentally suturing the superficial femoral nerve which relies in the subcutaneous tissue between TFL and Sa.

Postoperative care is unaffected by the approach utilised; full weight bearing is allowed at day 1 postoperatively and hospital discharge from day 3 or 4.

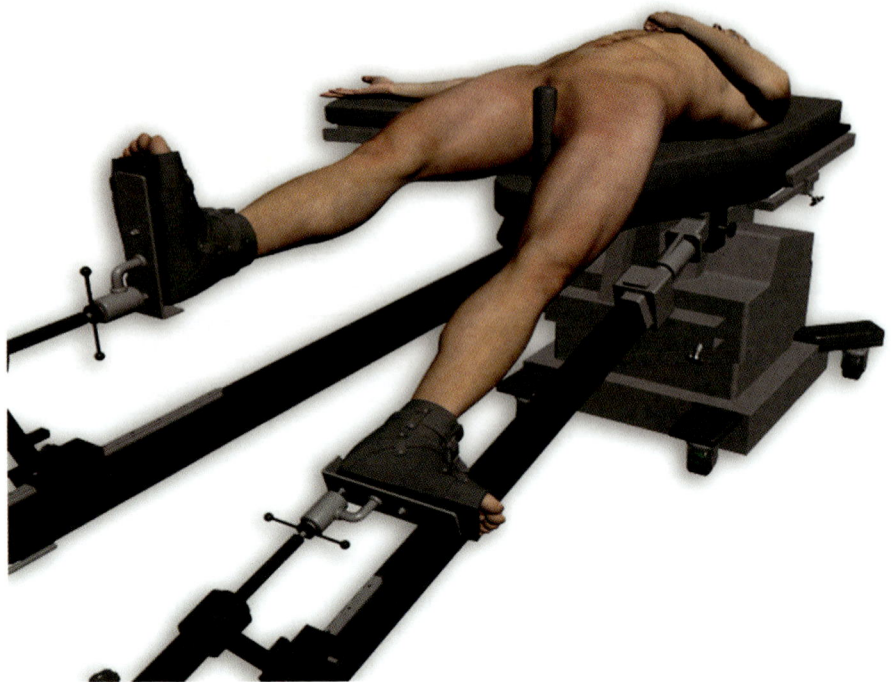

Fig. 10.4

Preliminary Series and Discussion

From 2002 to the end of 2004, we resurfaced 61 hips in 36 males and 25 females with either Conserve Plus (Wright Medical) or ASR (DePuy). The mean age of our patients was 43 year (25–53). Half the cases were due to juvenile degenerative arthritis and the rest mainly low-volume necrosis and posttrauma arthritis.

All of them were operated upon by the anterior approach as described above.

We have observed no significant early postoperative complications.

One patient presented with a secondary femoral neck fracture at 11 months post-operatively with a suspected low-grade infection. A THR was performed in a two-stage procedure.

The 60 other cases were prospectively followed up; all of them have been examined clinically and radiologically at 3–24 months.

Except for one patient who had unexplained pain at 12 months postop, all of them have a good or excellent clinical result with PMA score 16–18 with no restriction of social or sport activities.

Radiologically, the anterior approach enabled us to obtain correct positioning of the implant, despite the well-documented steep learning curves of this procedure.

All acetabular components were correctly placed; two femoral components were malpositioned, one with more than 20° of valgus from the neck axis and the other having 10° of varus. All the other cases were in between 0° and 10° of valgus.

Up to date, no late complications such as dislocation, heterotopic ossification, neck atrophy or implant bone fixation failure have been observed.

Discussion

This very short prospective series involving just two types of implant does not allow any conclusion to be made about resurfacing concept: We have a favourable initial impression but as yet no answers regarding uncemented fixation, the prevention of bone trabecular modification, the incidence of metal ion release and so on.

On the other hand, the anterior approach performed on an efficient orthopaedic table seems to be recommendable. The only absolute contraindications are resurfacing combined with femoral osteotomy or cases where simultaneous metalwork removal is required.

In all other cases, the advantages of this approach include:

- A sound anatomical basis, with all bone, muscles and tendons left intact
- A complete respect of the head and neck vascularisation
- Adaptability to all kind of implants (resurfacing or THR)
- Easily extendable where necessary
- Lack of iatrogenic complications
- Immediate rehabilitation and full weight bearing
- Cosmesis

So, for the marriage of resurfacing and a minimally invasive anterior approach, we have only great hopes for the implant but a complete and unrestricted faith in the approach!

References

1. Daniel J, Pynsent PB, McMinn DJ (2004) Metal-on-metal resurfacing of the hip in patients under the age of 55 years with osteoarthritis. J Bone Joint Surg Br 86(2):177–184
2. Judet TH, Siguier M, Brumpt B, Siguier TH, Piriou P (2005) Voie d'abord anterieure et prothèse de hanche de première intention. In: Puget J (ed) Prothèse totale de hanche. Les choix, Monographie de la SOFCOT. Elsevier, Paris
3. Siguier T, Siguier M, Brumpt B (2004) Mini-incision anterior approach does not increase dislocation rate: a study of 1037 total hip replacements. Clin Orthop Relat Res 426:164–173
4. Treacy RB, McBryde CW, Pynsent PB (2005) Birmingham hip resurfacing arthroplasty. A minimum follow-up of five years. J Bone Joint Surg Br 87(2):167–170

Chapter 11
Surgical Technique in Hip Resurfacing: Minimally Invasive Surgery with Posterior Approach

Michael Menge

Abstract Resurfacing of the hip with metal-on-metal devices is becoming more and more popular in younger patients. As the preserved femoral head interferes with the preparation of the socket, the standard approach needs longer incisions. This chapter describes a lesser invasive technique in hip resurfacing with posterior approach. Compared to the posterior and lateral standard techniques, the minimal dorsal approach needs an incision of around 10 cm, depending on the anatomical conditions; shortens the duration of the operation; decreases blood loss and the incidence of complications; and has high patient satisfaction. This technique therefore is recommended to surgeons who are familiar with the procedure of resurfacing with the dorsal approach.

Keywords Hip resurfacing • Posterior approach • Metal on metal device

Introduction

In 1991, Derek McMinn [1] introduced metal-on-metal resurfacing of the hip, and his final implant BHR became available in 1996. In 1999, we started to use this implant in our younger patients, and the midterm results were very promising [2–4]. According to the experience of McMinn, we used the dorsal approach for resurfacing. With growing experience and considering the tendencies to

M. Menge
Orthopädische Abteilung,
St. Marienkrankenhaus,
Salzburger Str. 15, Ludwigshafen D 67067, Germany
e-mail: michael.menge@st-marienkrankenhaus.de

D.G. Poitout, H. Judet (eds.), *Mini-Invasive Surgery of the Hip*,
DOI 10.1007/978-2-287-79931-0_11, © Springer France 2014

minimal invasive surgery, we tried to minimise the surgical trauma by reducing the extent of anatomical preparation without the necessity of special instrumentation or computerised navigation methods. The objective was not to obtain a cosmetically pleasing small scar but lesser invasive disruption of functional tissue, shorter time of exposition of the wound, less blood loss, and fewer complications. Since 2 years, the minimal invasive surgical dorsal approach proved to be superior to the dorsal and lateral standard approach and can be recommended to surgeons familiar with resurfacing procedures and the techniques of the dorsal approach.

Materials and Methods

Between 1999 and 2005, we performed more than 1,200 resurfacing procedures of the hip with different implants (BHR™, Cormet 2000™, ASR™, Durom™, Icon™, Bionik™, and Adept™). With growing experience, the rate of complications clearly decreased; the rate of early neck fractures diminished from 2.5 % in the beginning to 0.7 % in the last 2 years, and there was no late fracture (avascular necrosis of the head) in the last 300 resurfacings. With experience, there was the question of the original long incision of about 30 cm is needed for the posterior approach, and we started to develop a smaller approach without using the lateral guide pin. Minimal invasive surgery is said to have advantages, but there may be a higher risk of disadvantages due to the restricted visual field and therefore an increased overall complication rate. In our experience, the minimal invasive approach proved to be as safe as the conventional long incision technique. As two surgeons of our staff still prefer the lateral approach in resurfacing, there is the possibility to compare the early results of the described minimal invasive posterior procedure for resurfacing of the hip to the standard dorsal and the standard lateral approaches.

In the described minimal invasive dorsal approach, no special instrumentation is needed besides the standard instruments of the supplier of the used implant. We use an 8–12 cm incision at the dorsal third of the trochanter major, depending on the anatomical conditions, especially to the diameter of the subcutaneous fat layer. Disruptions of muscular structures cannot be avoided; the fibres of the greater gluteus muscle have to be split blunt, and the tendons of the piriformis muscle and the small external rotators have to be cut at the insertion at the greater trochanter and to be reaffixed after implantation of the prosthesis. Usually there is no bleeding from the dorsal circumflex artery, but there might be a violation of a smaller branch when detaching the upper portion of the quadratus femoris muscle in order to expose the base of the femoral neck. As with the short incision, there is no room for special gauges for positioning the axis of the cup; navigation has to be performed "by eye" and proved to be as exact as needed. The positioning of the acetabular socket has to consider the anatomical orientation as marked by the rim of the natural acetabulum with respect to pathological alterations by osteophytes.

The operation is mostly performed with spinal anaesthesia. During the procedure, there is no substantial blood loss, so drains are not necessary. We only use a plaster (Tegaderm™) staying for 5 days and then prefer open wound healing. As we have to use heparin in Germany for prevention of DVT to avoid legal complications, there will be considerable hidden blood loss in the days following mobilisation, but there is no need of preoperative haemodilution or transfusion. Walking with two sticks is allowed from the first day, stair climbing will be trained from the fourth day on and according to the conditions of the German DRG system, and the patient will be discharged after 7–10 days, depending on his convalescence. The patient is instructed to use crutches out of his accommodation for 6 weeks and to avoid exercises to "strengthen" the muscles.

Steps of the Procedure

The steps of the minimal invasive implantation of a resurfacing device are shown for the Adept™ hip, but there are only minimal differences to other products. There is no need for special reamers or other particular designed instruments.

1. The patient is placed on the side and fixed by holding devices; a foam tunnel is useful to place the leg over the healthy one below (Fig. 11.1). In the posterior approach, both components have to be placed by a single incision. With the hip to be operated in 45° flexion, the cut is performed at the dorsal third of the greater trochanter.
2. The tendon of the greater gluteal muscle is split sharply, and then the muscle fibres are divided bluntly with a scissor or with hooks. The trochanteric bursa is sharply split to be sutured at the end of the operation to adapt the muscle fibres of the proximal part of the quadratus muscle.
3. Now the palpating finger can find the gap between the posterior rim of the medial gluteus and the capsule of the hip joint. The sciatic nerve usually is palpable more dorsal; there is no need of exposing the nerve. Usually the tendon of the piriformis muscle can be felt easily. Mostly there is only one tendon but sometime one can expose the separate tendons of the gemelli and obturator muscles (Fig. 11.2).
4. A long curved Hohmann retractor exposes the capsule of the joint. Sometimes it is useful to separate some fibres of the gluteus minimus muscle from the capsule by means of a rasp.
5. The external rotators tendon is fixed by a suture and then detached from the greater trochanter.
6. In few cases, the distinct muscular structures of the small external rotators can be found at the insertion area of the greater trochanter.
7. Now the capsule can be split laterally and then from distal to the dorsal neck. Slight internal rotation facilitates the detaching of the dorsal capsule.
8. The hip is dislocated by internal rotation and flexion of the leg to 90°. The two-pronged Hohmann retractor is carefully inserted beneath the femoral head without violating soft tissue structures at the dorsal area of the joint.

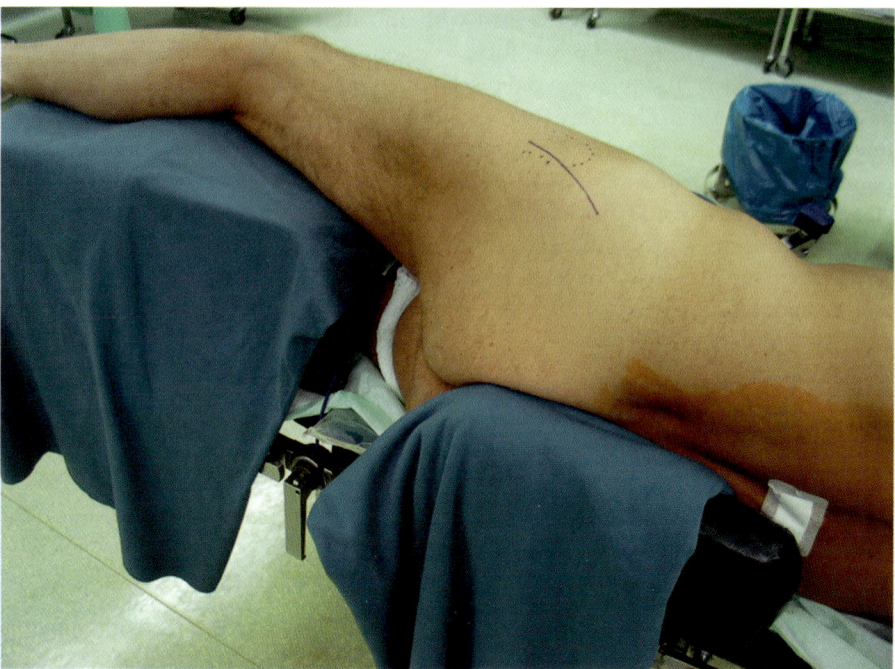

Fig. 11.1

9. When splitting the proximal base of the quadratus muscle, sometimes a branch of the dorsal circumflex artery may be violated and must be coagulated. With adduction, internal rotation, and flexion, the neck can easily be exposed. This is very important, as the neck has to be seen clearly from the posterior and proximal aspect. Remove the long curved Hohmann and hoist the femoral head by the two-pronged Hohmann retractor above the skin level. Two Hohmann retractors expose the distal femoral neck and the greater trochanter. Now the femoral neck should be exposed sufficiently to allow the determination of the axis of the neck and its projection to the femoral head (Fig. 11.3).

10. In minimal invasive resurfacing, the head must be prepared first. In cases of doubt regarding the sizes of the implants, prepare the head one size bigger than planned by the templates. It is easy to reduce the head size after implanting the smaller acetabular socket. Usually there is no room for navigation aids, but with the hemispherical templates for the neck, it is possible to project and to mark the axis of the femoral neck on the head. The instrumentation shown is provided with the Adept implant, but the instruments are identical in the BHR™, the Cormet 2000™, the Icon™, and other implants.

11. The midline axis of the neck is templated by a smaller gauge inserted from above. It should fit tightly as to mark the centre of the neck.

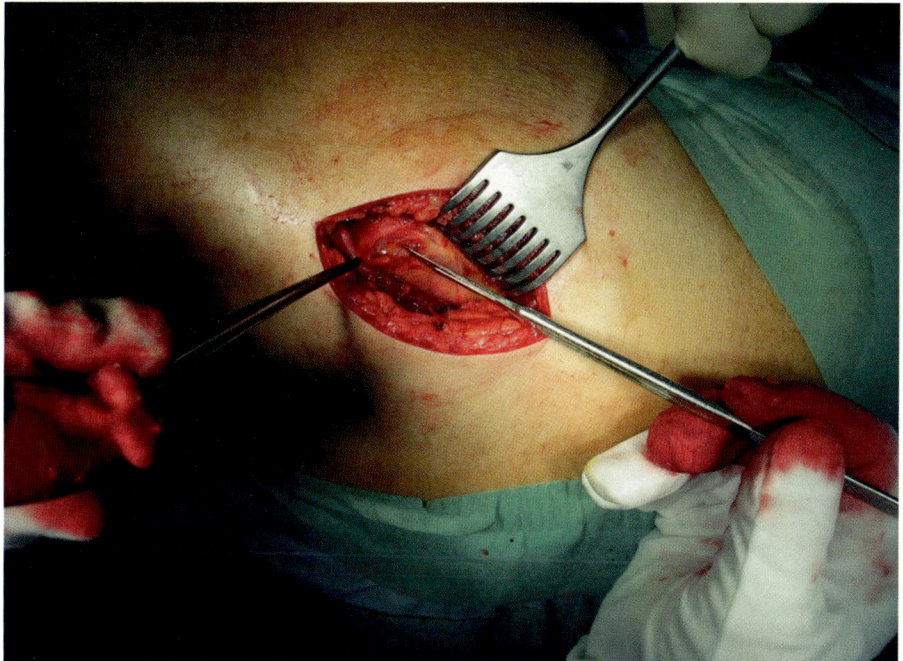

Fig. 11.2

12. As the cup should be positioned in neutral to slight valgus direction, the entrance of the guidewire should be positioned a little bit above the projected centre of the neck axis as preoperatively planned with the templates in the x-ray. The neck gauge should ensure not to notch the femoral neck with the cylindrical reamer.
13. Even in implants where the instrumentation does not provide suitable gauges, the guide pin can be positioned with a centring device (Durom™).
14. The appropriate drill overdrills the guide pin. The surgeons and his assistant should control the direction of the guidewire in both dimensions.
15. Now the axis may be controlled again and the cylindrical resection can be performed. Take care not to violate the dorsal skin by the reamer and not to notch the lateral base of the neck (Fig. 11.4).
16. Figure 11.4 demonstrates the removal of the resected cylinder.
17. After the cylindrical resection, the removal of the tip of the head has to be performed. To prevent early neck fracture, the cup has to cover the reamed head completely. Therefore, it is safer to resect enough of the head to ensure complete covering. Take care not to prolong the head as this might raise the risk of neck fracture. It is better to reconstruct the offset by placing the acetabular implant more laterally.

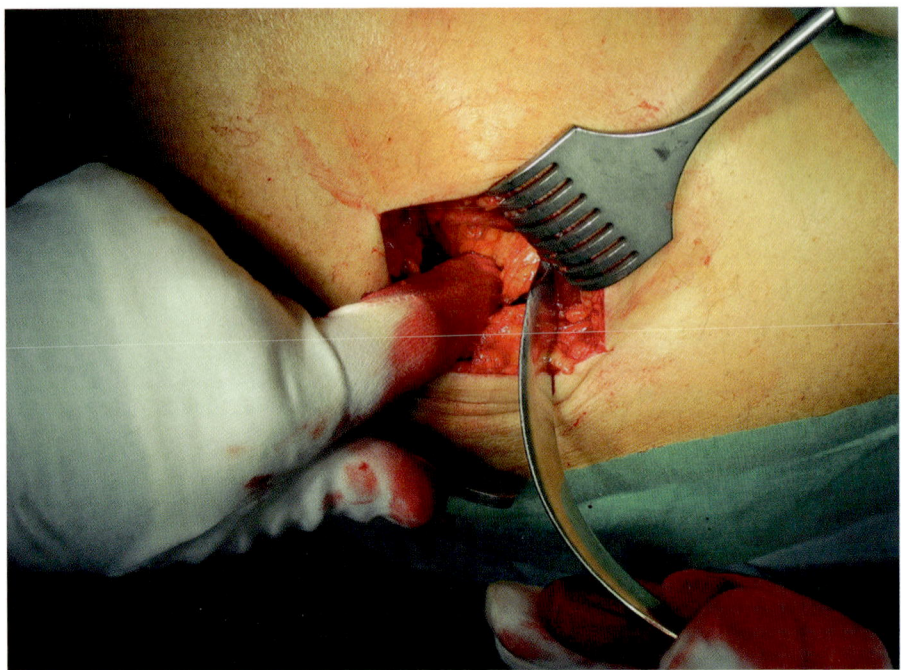

Fig. 11.3

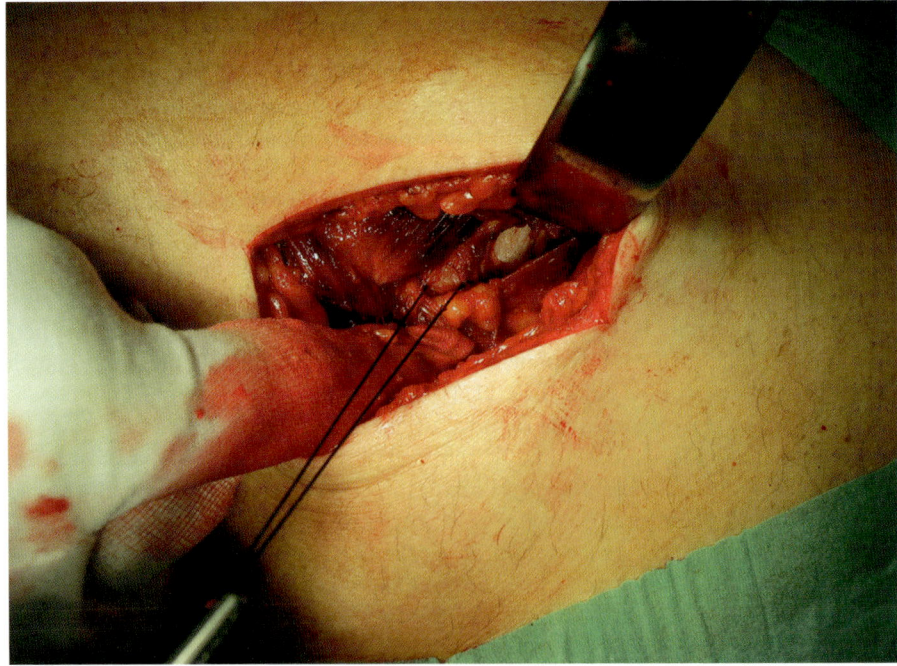

Fig. 11.4

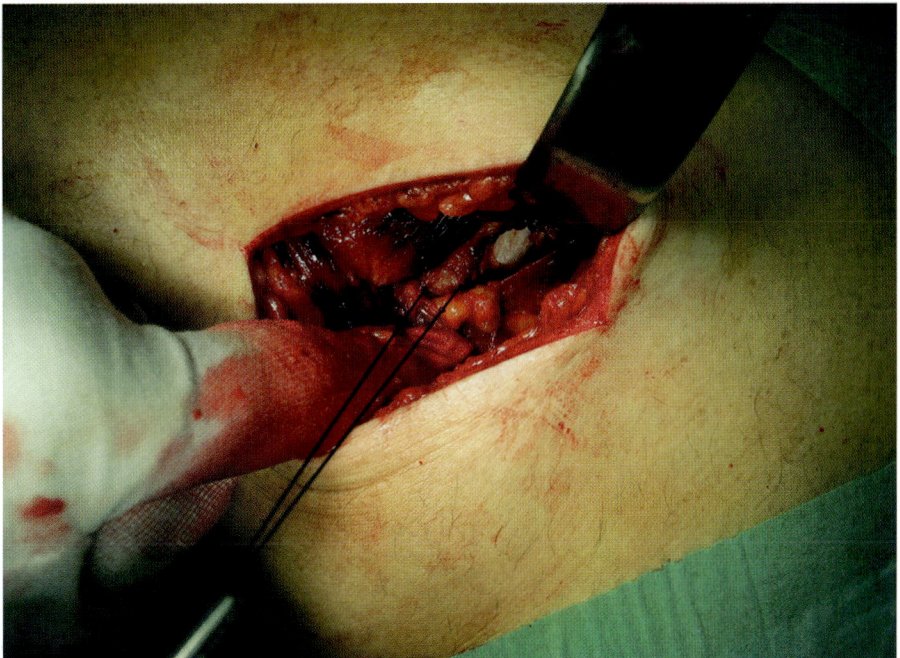

Fig. 11.5

18. Finally, the chamfer cut is performed. In the ASR™ system, the head resection is performed in one step (seen from distally).
19. Now the resection at the head of the femur is completed, and the head is small enough not to interfere with the preparation of the acetabulum.
20. To expose the acetabulum, the femoral head has to be shifted anterior and crani-ally. For safety of the soft tissue and the neurovascular structures, the cave of the acetabulum has to be palpated and the soft tissue smoothly is forced dorsally.
21. Place a long curved Hohmann under the neck of femur to the pelvic rim just above the insertion of the long head of the rectus muscle. Thus, the ventral neurovascular structures are far from the tip of the retractor and the acetabulum is best exposed. A blunt Hohmann retractor is positioned in the obturator fora-men and may be kept in position with a separated compress and a clamp to the cover of the leg. A Steinmann retractor in the ischium can be used to visualise the dorsal rim of the acetabulum.
22. After resecting the capsule and the limbus, the acetabulum can be overseen completely.
23. Now the acetabulum is reamed carefully to the guidelines of the manufac-turer of the implant (Fig. 11.5). The subchondral bone should be preserved as possible. When the subchondral sclerotic bone is preserved, the acetabulum should be underreamed about 1 mm, in cancellous bone about 2 mm. Now the final decision for the sizes of the implant is made. As the range of movement

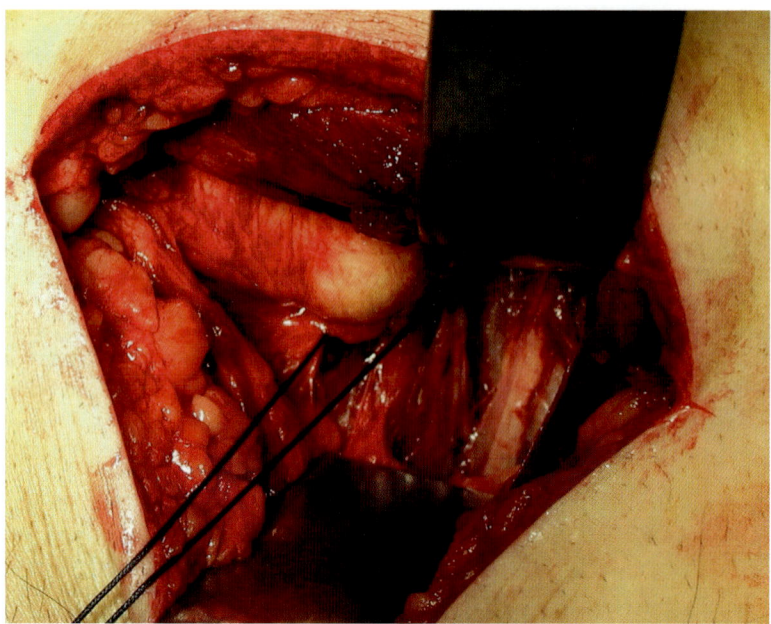

Fig. 11.6

in a resurfacing is inferior to a replacement with smaller neck, the socket
should get enough anteversion and more inclination than in replacement
procedures.

24. Figure 11.5 shows the aspect after reaming of the acetabulum.
25. Most manufacturers provide straight impactors that will do very well. In obese
    patients, the incision must give enough room distally.
26. In case of the Adept™ instrumentation, a double curved impactor facilitates the
    insertion of the socket.
27. The head is exposed again and the size in case reduced. We avoid any anchoring
    holes for the bone cement and only clean the surface by means of a jet lavage.
    For cups with press fit, we prefer low-viscosity cement to avoid big cement lay-
    ers preventing proper seating. A suction system may be applied to the greater
    trochanter to prevent invasion of the bone marrow into the vascular system.
28. The inner wall of the cup is covered with a thin layer of bone cement.
29. The cup is impacted properly. Most systems will provide a gauge to mark the
    point of correct seating (Fig. 11.6).
30. After cleansing of the wound, the hip is set and the wound should be cleaned by
    a pulse lavage. Take care not to entrap soft tissue between socket and cup.
31. The external rotators are refixed to the greater trochanter.
32. The same case as in Fig. 11.2 after refixation of the rotator group. Suture of the
    different layers (including the bursa) and wound closure as usual.

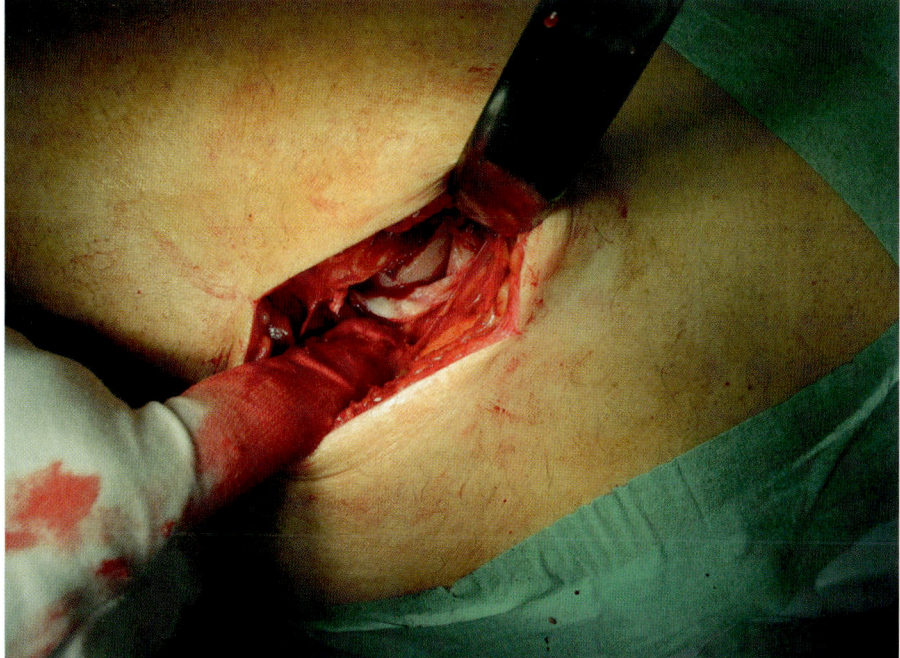

Fig. 11.7

33. After closing of the wound, a cosmetically pleasing short wound is obtained as a side effect (Fig. 11.7).
34. Typical aspect of the wound at discharge (sixth day postoperatively).

Results

The described technique was used by the author in more than 150 cases and now is used routinely. The advantage for the patient is a shorter operation time: Mean time between cut and suture of the skin was 54 (45–80) min, as in the original technique described by McMinn was 62 (55–80) min. There is no need for a drain, and there-fore, there will be no secretion of the drain holes in the course. No patient needed transfusion, the maximal drop of haemoglobin (Hb) was 3.6 g% at the eighth day postoperatively, and at the time of discharge, the Hb concentration was above 11 g%. Preoperative haemodilution will no longer be used for patients planned for MIS. With minimal invasive resurfacing, there was no infection, no wound healing disturbance, no nerve injury that far, and no dislocation. After the operation, the patients performed very well, and the time of hospitalisation (mean, 9.3 days) was shorter than after conventional technique (mean, 10.9 days). As expected, men left the hospital earlier than women (8.5 versus 10.3 days).

In patients with conventional lateral approach, the mean operation time was 97 (70–145) min from cut to suture; the blood loss was much higher, in mean 5.5 g% Hb at the third day and 4.7 g% Hb at the eighth day postoperatively. Eighteen percent of these patients needed transfusion. There were more complications in the group with lateral approach including dislocations, nerve injuries, and septic complications.

The comparison to the McMinn standard approach (dorsal, about 30 cm) was difficult: The mean operation time was about 62 min and all the patients underwent preoperative haemodilution. With autotransfusion, the preoperative Hb was 13.6 g%, and the maximum decrease in Hb was measured at the third day with −2.6 g%; at discharge, both groups had a mean Hb of 11 g%.

For the minimal invasive technique from the dorsal approach, there might be the problem of orientation and navigation as there are no tools for the beginner to estimate the axis of the guidewire and therefore for the stem of the cup. As was shown in the pictures in the technique section, it is inevitable to get clear site of the neck of the femur and to place the guidewire exactly. Then the deviation from the ideal axis is neglectable. So the minimal invasive technique should be recommended only to surgeons familiar with the dorsal approach and the technique of estimating the axis of the femoral neck.

Discussion

Less and minimal invasive surgical techniques may give shorter skin incisions, but indubitably, it is more important to maintain anatomic structure's integrity. If it is possible to reduce dissecting of any anatomical structures that is not absolutely necessary, there will be a chance to meet the needs of the patient: less pain, shorter stay in hospital, and faster recovery. On the other side, there might be the risk of malposition of the implant, neurovascular complications, and injury to skin and soft tissue by excessive retraction of the skin and pressure of the instruments because of the restricted visual field.

As shown in the technical section, a minimised dorsal approach will give excellent oversight to all of the important landmarks. Additional instruments for control of the direction of the guidewire into the head of the femur cannot be used, so theoretically there is a possibility of missing the exact axis of the femoral neck. In cases of extremely contract joints, the surgeon has to decide whether he has to switch to a standard procedure.

There is no need for special instruments besides the two-pronged and the long curved Hohmann retractors shown in Fig. 11.8. The minimal invasive technique is usable not only in young, thin, healthy, and motivated patients but now is standard procedure in most resurfacing procedures with the mentioned seven products. In obese patients, the skin incision has to be longer than 10 cm but not as long as in the standard procedure.

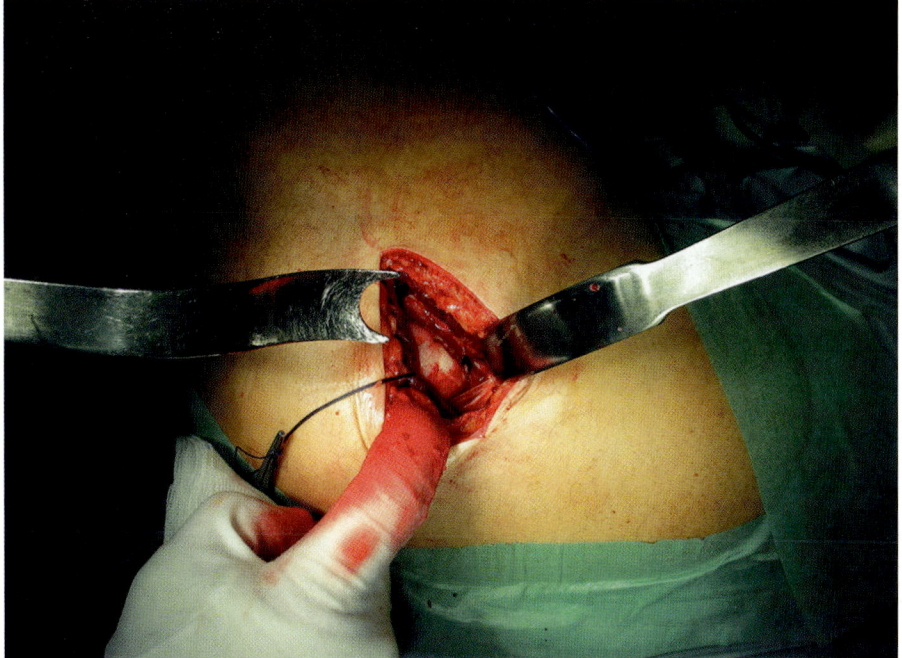

Fig. 11.8

Conclusion

According to the guidelines of the American Association of Hip and Knee Surgeons [5], less invasive hip replacement surgery "has not validated for same or better long-term results, with shorter and less painful recovery". In our series of more than 1,200 resurfacings of the hip within the last 6 years [4], we have gathered some experience with the surgical technique, and for the experienced surgeon, it seems to be unnecessary to expose and to detach anatomical structures not needed for the goal of the procedure. As we have learned by minimising the exposition of the hip from the dorsal approach, it will be easily be possible to perform the resurfacing procedure with normal instruments and with optimal visibility of all needed anatomical landmarks and vital structures. The midterm (up to 2 years) results of the minimal invasive resurfacings are identical to those after standard approach, but there is considerable benefit besides improved cosmesis: The duration of the operation is shorter (13–45 %), there is significant lesser blood loss, rehabilitation is faster, and the patient may leave the hospital earlier. We did not evaluate the differences in postoperative pain after standard or minimal invasive procedure, but our impression is that most patients did discontinue antiphlogistic medication earlier after minimal invasive surgery. There was no report of thromboembolism, nerve damage, or infection, and the patients expressed a high grade of satisfaction [1].

As a summary, we have to state that the described technique of minimal invasive resurfacing arthroplasty of the hip joint from a posterior approach should be seen only as an optimised standard technique. We use seven different standard implants for resurfacing with standard instrumentation. The difference to the "contemporary incisions" is only the familiarity with the procedure of resurfacing and the intention to avoid unnecessary detachments and incisions. So we can recommend the described procedure of minimal invasive resurfacing surgery from the posterior approach to those surgeons who are generally familiar with resurfacing procedures. The patient will profit from shorter hospitalisation, faster recovery, and a lesser rate of complications. At least, he will enjoy of a cosmetically shorter incision.

References

1. McMinn D, Treacy R, Lin K, Pynsent P (1996) Metal-on-metal surface replacement of the hip. Clin Orthop Relat Res (329 Suppl):S89–98
2. Menge M (2003) Aktueller Stand der Hüftendoprothetik mit proximalen knochensparenden Alloplastiken. Orthop Prax 39:555–563
3. Menge M (2004) Metal on metal in resurfacing arthroplasty: risks or benefits? In: Lazennec JY, Dietrich M (eds) Bioceramics in joint arthroplasty. 9th Biolox symposium, proceedings. Steinkopff, Darmstadt, pp 111–117
4. Menge M (2005) Oberflächenersatz am Hüftgelenk – 6-Jahres-Erfahrungen mit der dritten Generation. Z Orthop 143:377–381
5. American Association of Hip and Knee Surgeons (2004) Minimally invasive and small incision joint replacement surgery: what surgeons should consider. www.aahks.org

Chapter 12
Navigation and the Square Angle Pointer in Hip Resurfacing

N. Szöke

Keywords Navigation • Hip resurfacing • Square angle pointer • Metal on metal bearings • D. McMinn arthroplasty

Introduction

Historically resurfacing arthroplasty with metal on polyethylene bearings (Wagner cup) has had high failure rates due to the tissue reaction from the high volumetric polyethylene wear. In our days, with advanced metal-on-metal bearings, the volumetric wear has been reduced, and resurfacing hip arthroplasty becomes a bone-conserving alternative to standard total hip arthroplasty in young and active patients [1].

Derek McMinn introduced the new generation of metal-on-metal resurfacing arthroplasty in 1991 [2].

We started in 1998 with hip resurfacing. Between 1998 and 2007, we performed more than 1,800 operations. Indications for resurfacing are mainly osteoarthritis, posttraumatic arthritis, femoral head osteonecrosis, slipped capital femoral epiphysis or dysplasia.

With growing evidence that performing hip and knee arthroplasy and spine surgery using navigation can lead to a more accurate surgical positioning of the components with when a conventional operating technique without navigation is used, it was on the hand to start with navigation also for resurfacing [3–6].

In the hospital, we use the imageless navigation system from BrainLab for the knee arthroplasty.

N. Szöke
Department für Endoprothetik, Eduardus Krankenhaus,
Custodis Str. 3-17, Köln D 50679, Germany
e-mail: nszoeke@yahoo.de

D.G. Poitout, H. Judet (eds.), *Mini-Invasive Surgery of the Hip*,
DOI 10.1007/978-2-287-79931-0_12, © Springer France 2014

After cadaver trials, we started using the VectorVision Hip SR software in our operating theatres from August 2005 for hip resurfacing [2].

The Operative Technique

A standard posterior approach is used in all patients, the skin incision measuring 8–15 cm, depending on the BMI of the patient. After splitting the gluteus maximus, the trochanteric bursa is cut and the piriformis tendon is visualised. Following this, the fibres of the gluteus minimus are separated from the capsule. The gemellus muscles and the obturator internus are cut. The capsule is opened circumferentially. The hip is then dislocated and the actual navigation begins.

The trochanter minor is visualised and the femur reference array is installed (Fig. 12.1). This is followed by the femoral shaft axis calculation where we first acquire the landmark points of the medial and lateral epicondyle (Fig. 12.2) and the landmark point of the piriformis fossa using the pointer.

Then the head-neck junction point is landmarked as well; this point is going to be used as a reference for the initial implant position (Fig. 12.3).

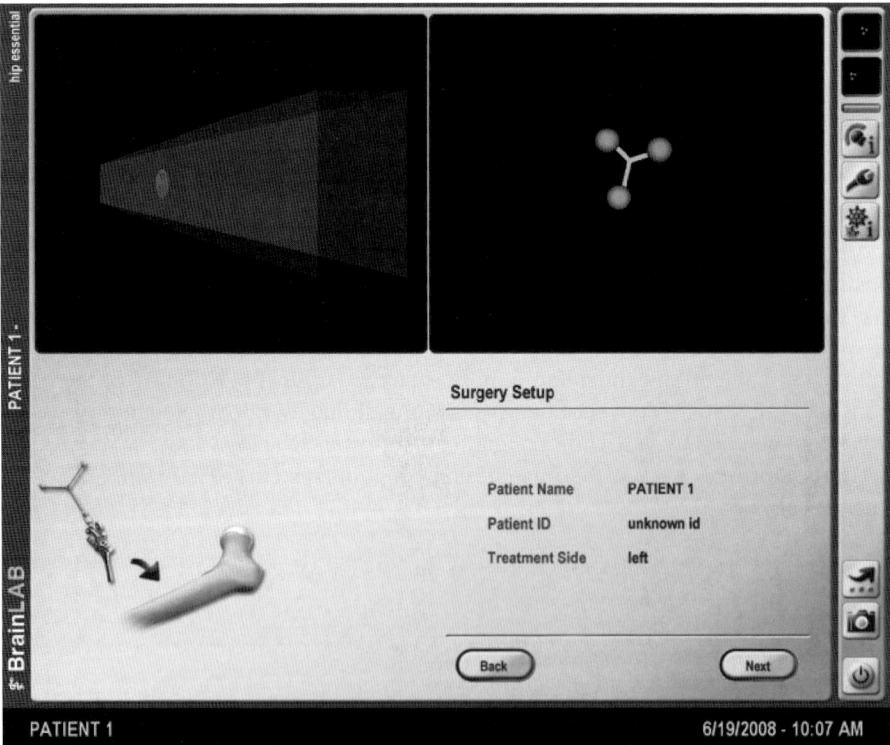

Fig. 12.1 Attachment of the reference arrays

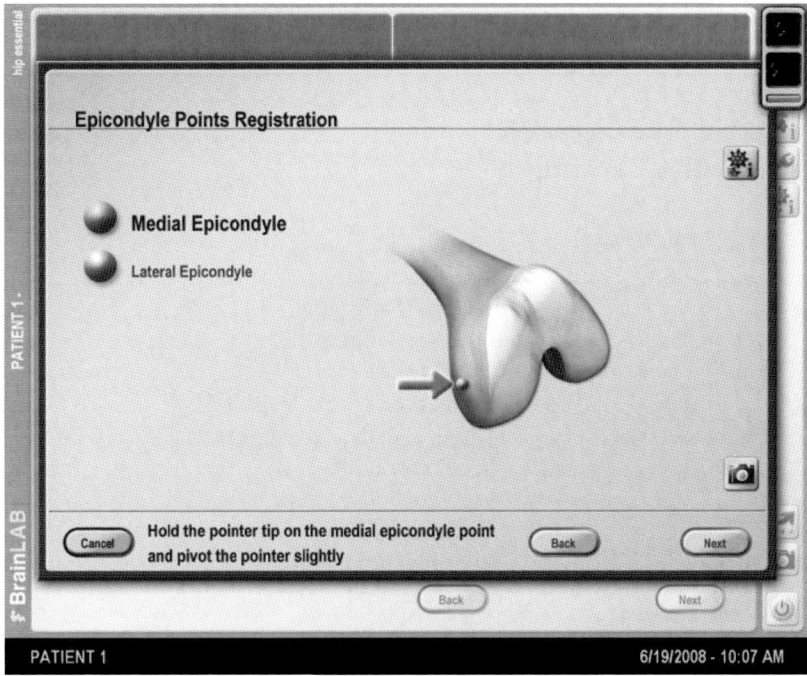

Fig. 12.2 Acquisition of the medial condyle point

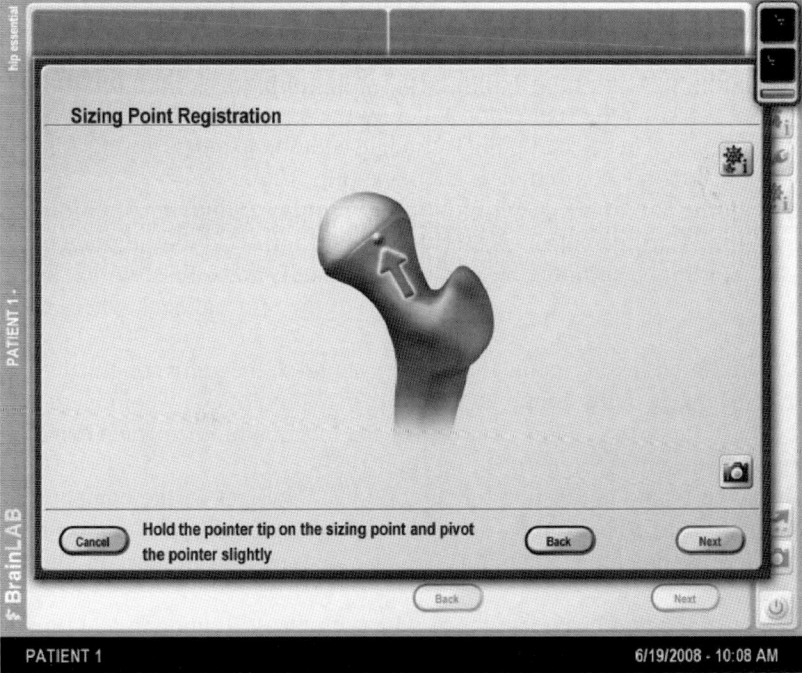

Fig. 12.3 Acquisition of the head-neck junction point

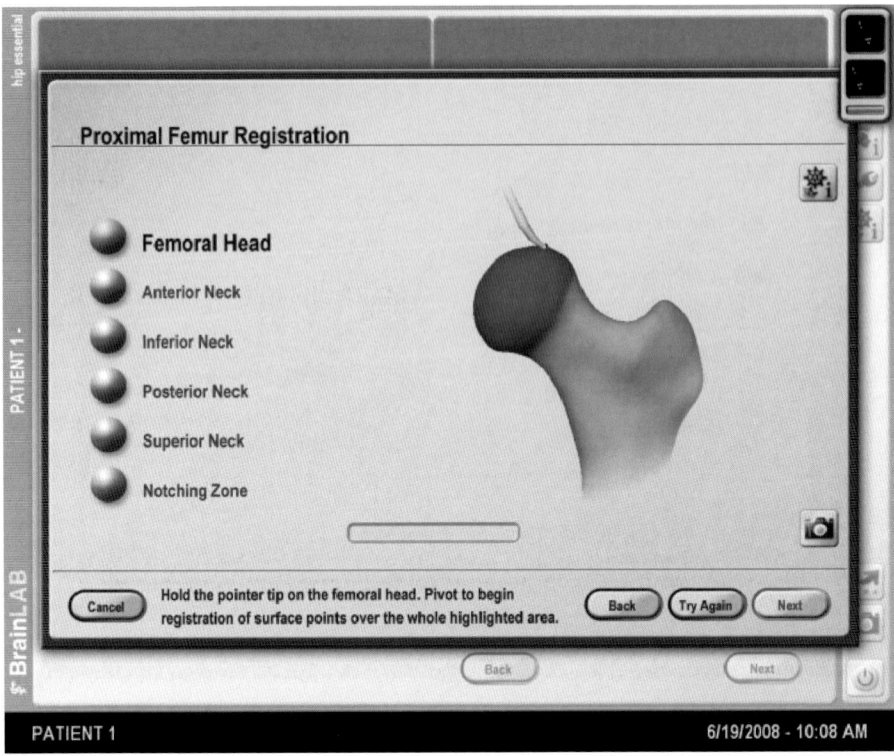

Fig. 12.4 Proximal femur registration

Now we work out the centre of rotation of the femoral head using the pointer to sample the femoral head. This point is used, in addition to the piriformis fossa point, to define the femoral axis and the axial plane (Fig. 12.4).

The calculation of the neck axis follows, making landmark points on the anterior (Fig. 12.5), superior, posterior and inferior neck. These points are also used to determine the notching zone. Additionally it is possible to define the superior notching zone, the most likely area of the femoral neck where notching occurs.

After all the necessary points have been acquired, the software creates a three-dimensional image of the femur, which has then to be verified by holding the pointer to the known landmarks. This assures that the location on the screen actually correlates with the actual pointer position (Fig. 12.6).

It is now possible to position the femoral head implant on the computer model and make very fine corrections in all three dimensions. Should this position the implant into a notching zone, this is indicated by red colour on the screen (Fig. 12.7).

It is now possible to navigate the K-wire with the drill guide in real time to the planned implant position (Fig. 12.8). With this, the navigation part of the operation is finished (8).

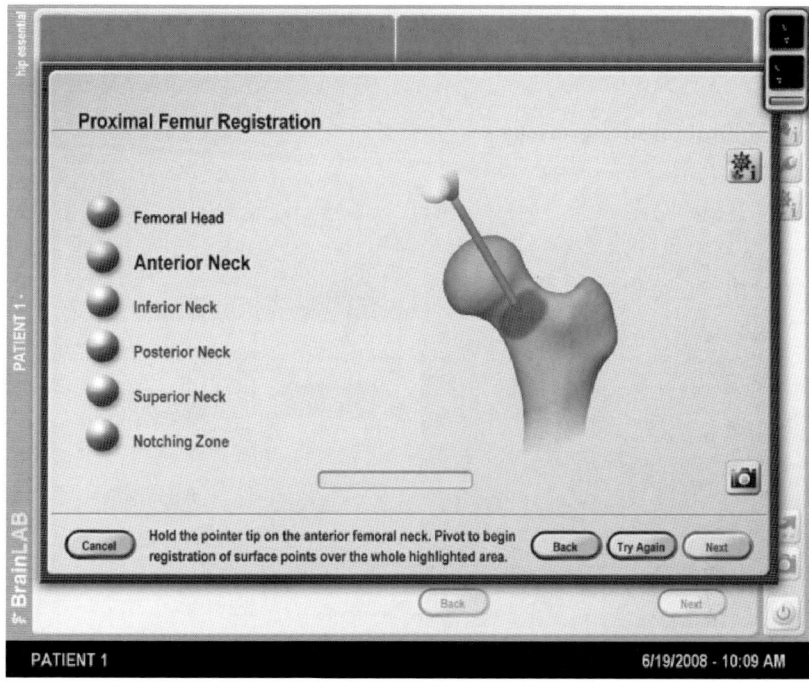

Fig. 12.5 Anterior neck registration

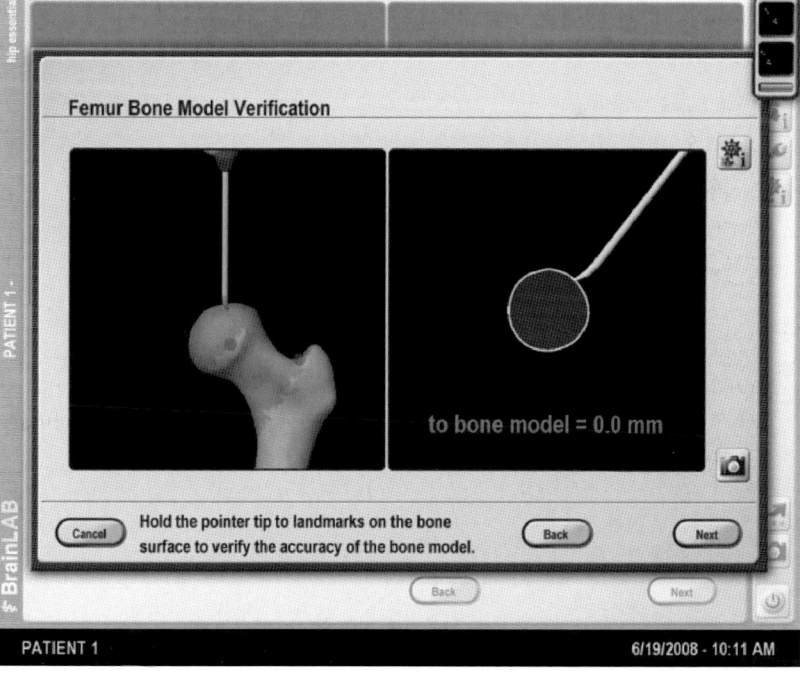

Fig. 12.6 Verification of femur model

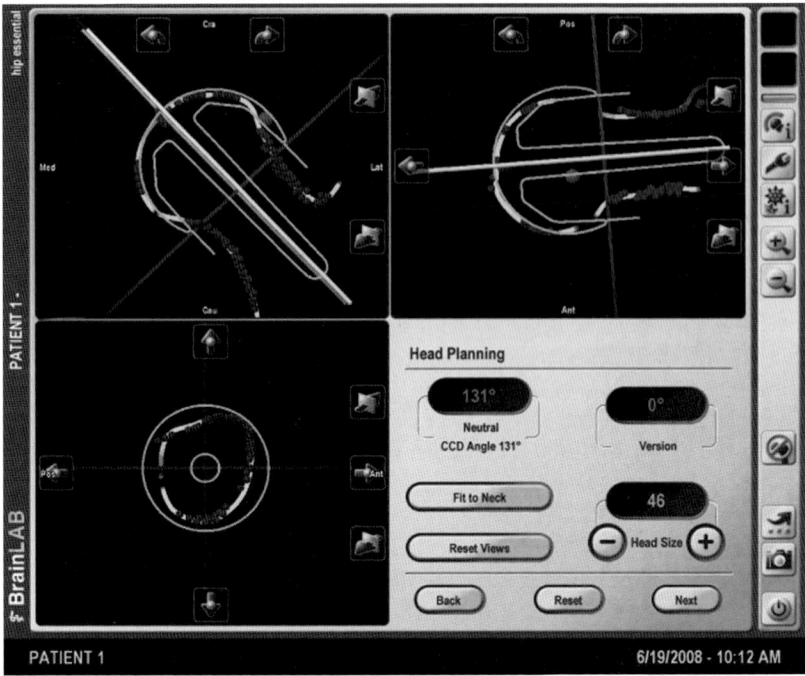

Fig. 12.7 Implant positioning

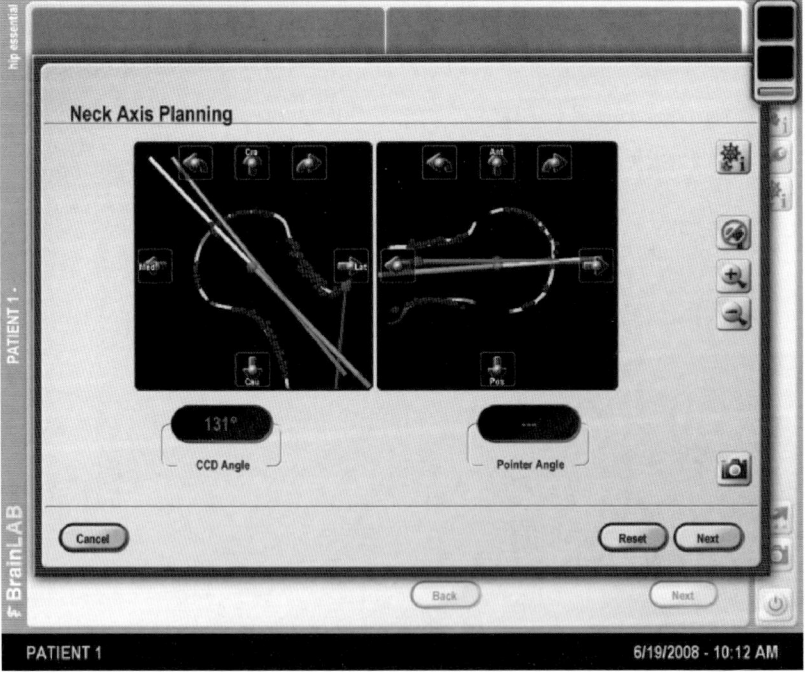

Fig. 12.8 Navigating the K-wire

Discussion

Hip resurfacing is a technically high demanding procedure with a long learning curve.

Freehand positioning with the mechanical jig technique is difficult, and it is hard to determine for the operating surgeon what the exact position of the implant is. That is why we started using navigation systems in 2005 with the BrainLab VectorVision Hip SR Software. With navigation, we are not confronted with intra-operative femoral neck notching, and it is easy to avoid varus malpositioning. However, our operating times have been increased by between 10 and 20 min using the straight pointer and the first version of the navigation software.

The main problem was for us to successfully landmark the right points on the anterior and also lateral part of the femoral neck with the long straight pointer (Fig. 12.9). This leads to the software showing us calculating errors in 20 % of our operations, causing us to abort the navigation and going back to conventional mechanical jig technique.

After the introduction of the square angle pointer (Fig. 12.10), which we had asked for to be introduced in order to avoid the problem of not being able to reach the right landmark points and us having switched to the newer VectorVision Hip SR 1.0 Software, we did not need extra operating time. Additionally we did not have to abort using the navigation software during any of the surgeries during which we used the square angle pointer, as no more calculating errors appeared.

Following this initial success, we have now started a prospective randomised study comparing the results of operations in which no navigation has been used with the results of those operations in which we used the new navigation software in connection with the square angle pointer.

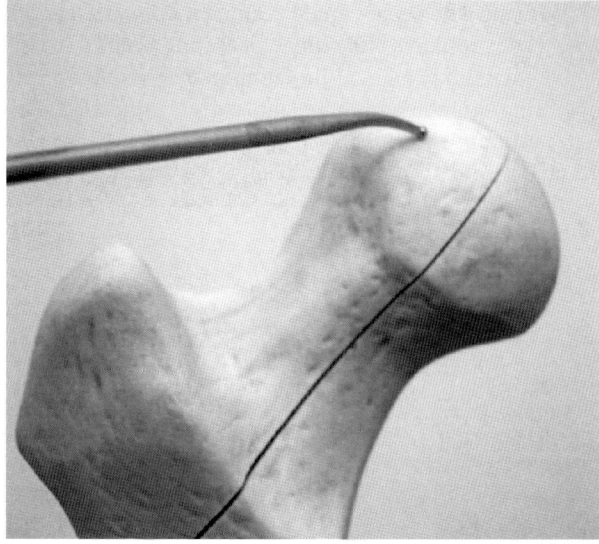

Fig. 12.9 Straight pointer

Fig. 12.10 Square pointer

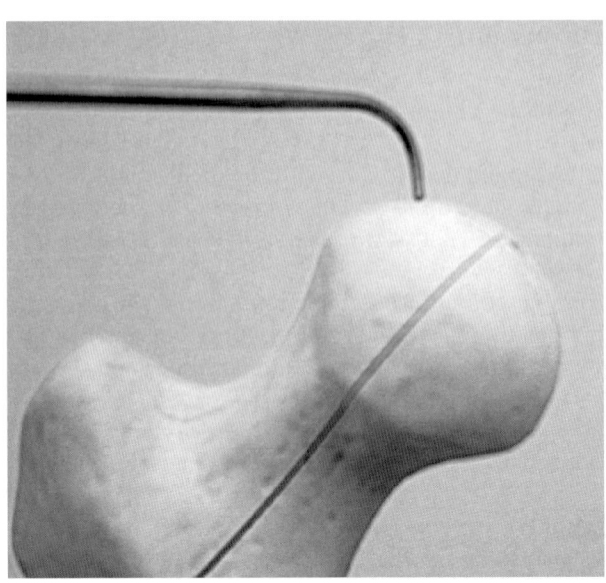

Conclusion

The accurate placement of the implant is very important in hip resurfacing in order to avoid notching and varus positioning of the head. Navigation with the straight pointer and earlier software allowed thorough three-dimensional intra-operative analysis, which enabled the surgeon to avoid femoral neck notching and ensured a better alignment of the femoral component with the frontal and sagittal planes. However, operating times have generally been increased, and the navigation part of some of the surgeries had to be aborted due to the previously mentioned problems.

With the new square angle pointer and the newer software, we were able to eliminate these problems and reduce operating times to what they were when we used the conventional mechanical jig technique. Navigation provides greater security to the operating surgeon and represents a great educational and training tool.

The future has to show if the necessary additional investment will bring better clinical results.

References

1. Daniel J, Pynsent PB, McMinn DJ (2004) Metal-on-metal resurfacing of the hip in patients under age of 55 years with osteoarthritis. J Bone Joint Surg Br 86(2):177–184
2. McMinn D, Treacy R, Lin K et al (1996) Metal-on-metal surface replacement of the hip. Clin Orthop Relat Res (329 Suppl):S89–98

3. Honl M et al (2003) Comparison of robot assisted and manual implantation of a primary total hip replacement. A prospective study. J Bone Joint Surg Am 85:1470–1478
4. Callaghan JJ, Liu SS, Warth LC (2006) Computer-assisted surgery: a wine before its time: in the affirmative. J Arthroplasty 21(4 Suppl):27–28
5. Amiot LP, Lang K, Putzier M et al (2000) Comparative results between conventional and computer-assisted pedicle screw installation in the thoracic, lumbar, and sacral spine. Spine 25:606–614
6. Sparmann M, Wolke B, Czupalla H et al (2003) Positioning of total knee arthroplasy with and without navigation support. A prospective, randomized study. J Bone Joint Surg Br 85: 830–835

Chapter 13
Navigated Modular Short-Stemmed Total Hip Arthroplasty by a Less Invasive Technique

Djordje Lazovic, Ferenc József Dunai, and Rasmus Zigan

Abstract Since 2004, we have been using a modular short-stemmed hip prosthesis with a less invasive anterolateral approach in 270 cases. The modified Watson-Jones (Br J Surg 23:787–808, 1936) approach allows the insertion of the hip prosthesis without detaching muscles. The modularity of the prosthesis offers the choice of different degrees of anteversion and CCD angles to restore hip biomechanics, which is simulated by the navigation system. We evaluated primary stability, ease of minimally invasive implantation and restoration of biomechanics. We found good functional results and a low complication rate, without any dislocation. The navigation helps to insert the cup more precisely and to restore the centre of rotation, leg length and offset. It suggests the best choice of modular neck to use and helps to predict and influence the safe range of motion. The emphasis is placed on the description of the surgical steps.

Keywords Surgical technique • Navigation • Total hip arthroplasty • Short-stemmed prosthesis • Modular neck • Minimal invasive surgery

Introduction

An increasing demand for less traumatic THA combined with a faster recovery time has led to bone and soft tissue preserving short-stemmed prostheses [1] and to minimally invasive surgical approaches with reduced blood loss, faster recovery time and safe primary stability for full weight bearing [2, 3].

D. Lazovic (✉) • F.J. Dunai • R. Zigan
Clinic for Orthopedics, Pius-Hospital Oldenburg,
Georgstrasse 12, Oldenburg D-26121, Germany
e-mail: djordje.lazovic@pius-hospital.de

D.G. Poitout, H. Judet (eds.), *Mini-Invasive Surgery of the Hip*,
DOI 10.1007/978-2-287-79931-0_13, © Springer France 2014

The need for joint stability and higher mobility after THA has led to navigated hip surgery together with the use of modular necks to restore hip biomechanics. Navigation has proved to be a useful tool to achieve more precise positioning of THA implants, which should improve their longevity and biomechanics [4]. The changes in biomechanics of the hip are visualised and can easily be influenced with a modular implant [5].

Short-stemmed hip implants are designed for cementless fixation in the proximal part of the femur [1]. The short-stemmed Metha hip prosthesis has a modular neck and can be implanted with the aid of THA navigation. To achieve primary stability, the prosthesis relies on multipoint contact in the femoral metaphysis. This forces the stem of the prosthesis into a nearly preset implant position, with only little variability, which can affect the biomechanics of the hip in terms of leg length and offset. The modular construction of the prosthesis decouples stem position from joint reconstruction. It enables the surgeon to influence joint geometry with greater variability and without compromising secure fixation in the femur [6]. The use of kinematic navigation technology supports the selection of modular implant components in order to optimise joint reconstruction and range of motion [5].

A correct surgical indication is a prerequisite for successful implantation of short-stemmed hip prostheses. In particular, the quality and shape of the bone must be considered. Unsuitable bone shapes include coxarthritis secondary to congenital dysplasia of the hip with extreme coxa valga, a short and wide femoral neck, pronounced coxa vara as well as previous surgery with gross deformation of the proximal femur. Osteoporosis can affect the primary stability of the implant and lead to subsidence or fractures.

Material and Methods

Patient Population

From November 2004 to March 2010, we have performed 270 hip arthroplasties using a short–stemmed implant. Patients for this procedure were selected according to age, bone quality and previous surgery. In our first series, we limited patient age to less than 50 years, but with more confidence in the implant, we have extended the age limit to 69 years, provided good bone quality could be assumed in active patients. Exclusion criteria included osteoporosis as well as previous surgery with gross changes of the anatomy of the proximal femur. On the basis of our good experience using navigation with standard THA, the cup was implanted routinely with the aid of navigation. Following a learning period, we started to insert the stem using navigation too, so that 210 short stems have been navigated. This leads to two groups, which are compared in the results.

Indications were primary coxarthritis in 43 %, secondary coxarthritis in dysplastic hips in 46 % and femoral head necrosis in 11 %. One-hundred and forty five patients were female and 125 male with a mean age of 50 years. One-hundred and eighteen left and 152 right hips were replaced. The body mass index (BMI) was slightly heavy with 27.1.

Implant Devices

The same device was used in all patients. The cup is a hemispherical titanium press-fit cup with a plasma spray coating (Plasmacup SC, BBraun Aesculap, Tuttlingen, Germany) and a ceramic insert (BIOLOX forte and BIOLOX delta). The cup implant used has three holes, which allow an additional fixation with bone screws.

The femoral prosthesis is a short-stemmed design for metaphyseal fixation with modular neck adapters (Metha, BBraun Aesculap, Tuttlingen, Germany). It offers the choice between different degrees of antetorsion ($-7.5°$, $0°$, $+7.5°$) and different CCD angles ($130°$, $135°$ and $140°$). For the nine different types of neck, the length could be adjusted by varying the length of the ceramic heads, i.e. short (-3.5 mm), medium (0 mm), long ($+3.5$ mm) or, in heads with a diameter of more than 32 mm, extra long ($+7$ mm). This leads to numerous possibilities to restore the desired biomechanics independent of the stem position. The femoral stem is inserted to optimally fit the proximal femur with its multipoint fixation that depends on the natural shape of the proximal femur, its antetorsion and the resection level of the neck. Primary fixation is by press fit; secondary fixation is secured by the proximal coating that allows bony ingrowth; the non-coated tip is only needed for primary fixation (Fig. 13.1).

Navigation System

We have been using an X-ray-free kinematic navigation system since 2001 (OrthoPilot, BBraun Aesculap, Tuttlingen, Germany), which has been developed and improved further in terms of software and hardware since then. The current technique employs passive rigid bodies whose position is detected by an infrared-emitting camera. The software allows control of the acetabular reamer and the final implant, taking into consideration inclination, anteversion, centre of rotation and depth for the cup. For the short-stemmed prosthesis, the femoral navigation was employed to control leg length, changes in offset and antetorsion and to predict the free range of motion in a safe zone to avoid dislocation. By providing this information, it helps to choose the right combination of modular neck and head out of the various possibilities.

Fig. 13.1 The short-stemmed Metha
prosthesis is coated on the proximal,
metaphyseal area, which supports bony
ingrowth and secondary stability. The tip is
smooth and is only needed for primary
stability. The neck is modular and can be
chosen with variable degrees of antetorsion
and CCD angles

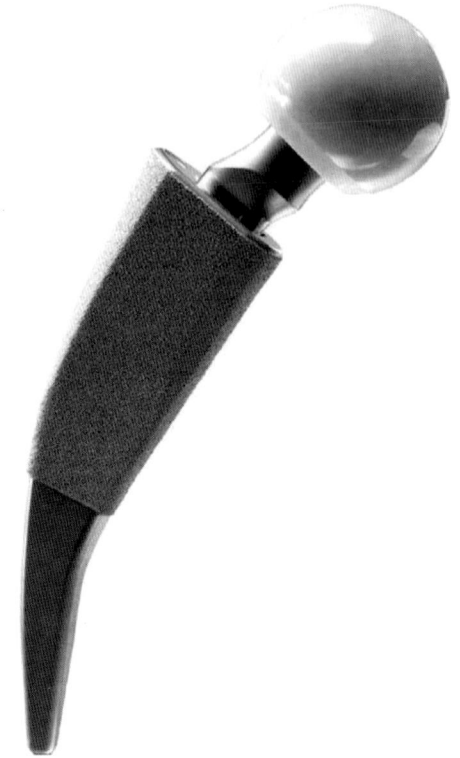

Surgical Technique

Patient Positioning and Draping

The patient is placed supine on a standard radiolucent table. The navigation
camera is placed on the contralateral side at the foot end of the table, at a distance of about 2 m. Prepping the operative field includes the ipsilateral iliac
crest. Draping allows free movement of the entire leg and free palpation of both
anterior superior iliac spines and the pubic symphysis. These landmarks are
needed to determine the pelvic plane on which the calculation of the acetabular
inclination and anteversion is based. Before starting the surgical approach to the
hip, the ipsilateral iliac spine is identified and a 5 mm stab incision is made on
the iliac crest about 4 cm dorsal to the anterior superior iliac spine. To avoid
later irritations of the scar, the skin is tensed over the iliac crest, so that the scar
will be caudal to the bone contour. A screw pin is fixed to the iliac crest on
which the rigid body is adapted. The anatomic landmarks are then recorded with
a pointer (Fig. 13.2).

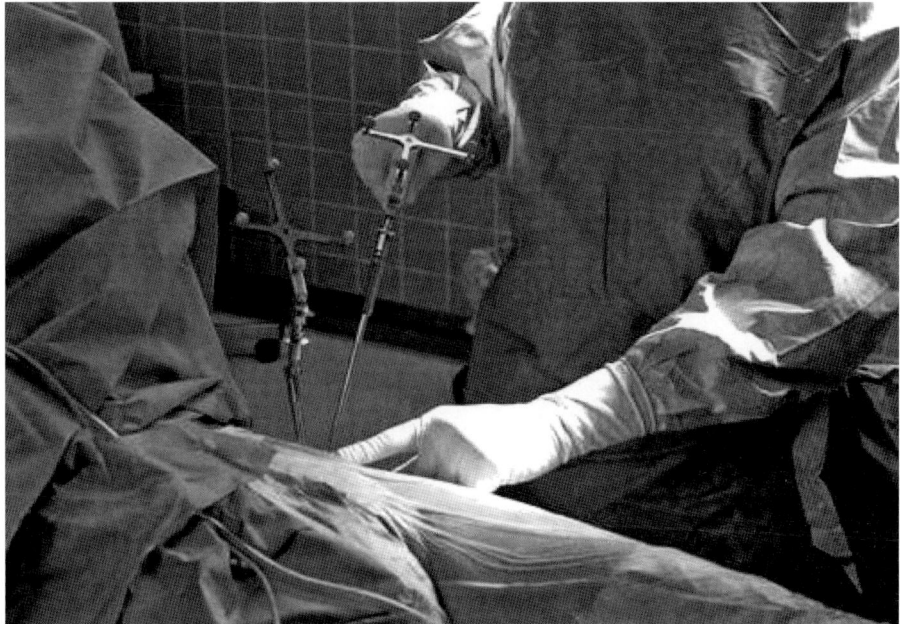

Fig. 13.2   After placing the rigid body in the iliac crest, the landmarks of the pelvis are palpated with a pointer to register the anterior pelvic plane

Surgical Approach

We have been using a modified and minimised anterolateral Watson-Jones approach [7]. The skin incision is about 8–10 cm long on the level of the anterior border of the greater trochanter. It extends from near the distal end of the greater trochanter to about 2–4 cm proximal of the tip of the trochanter. The fascia lata is displayed and split. In case of a trochanteric bursitis, the bursa is resected. The space between the vastus lateralis muscle and the gluteus medius is identified and split bluntly, a vessel occurring regularly in this place is cauterised. Then the capsule is exposed using two blunt curved Hohmann retractors, which are placed around the neck, and one pointed wide-bladed Hohmann retractor which is placed over the anterior rim of the pelvis. An oblique incision is made over the femoral neck from the medial proximal pelvic attachment of the capsule to the lateral distal femoral attachment. Two additional parallel incisions complete the Z-shaped opening of the capsule. The extent of this incision should allow dislocation of the femoral head, but can be extended to the lesser trochanter in case of contractures.

Before dislocating the hip, biomechanical data must be collected for the navigation system. A C-shaped clamp for the fixation of the femoral rigid body is

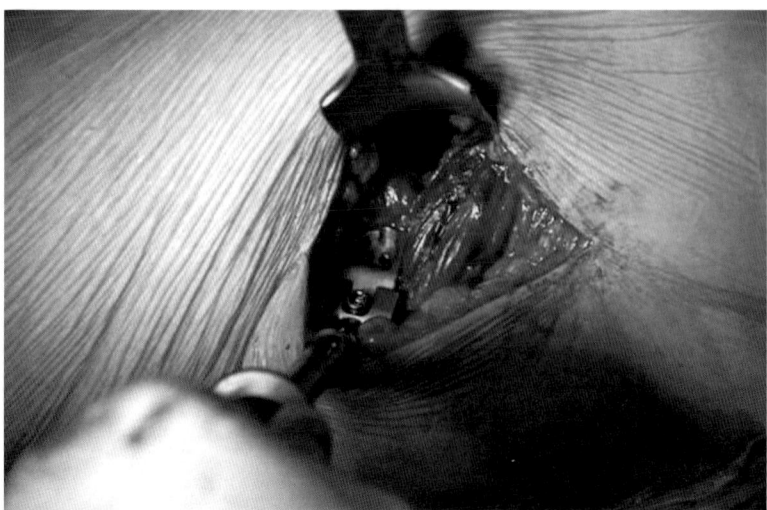

Fig. 13.3 A C-shaped clamp is placed on the femur, distal to the insertion of the gluteus muscle. The rigid body can be fixed and detached by a bayonet connection

placed on the femur slightly distal to the greater trochanter at the transition to the diaphysis of the femur. Placement of the clamp is facilitated by abducting the leg and rotating it slightly inward. Lately, we have been using a clamp holding device, which makes positioning more comfortable. First, we record the neutral position of the extended leg and then the centre of the patella and the ankle joint, both of which are recorded with the knee flexed at 90°. These data allow calculating the axis of the femur and the antetorsion of the femoral neck. To continue surgery, the rigid body can be removed from the clamp by a bayonet connection (Figs. 13.3 and 13.4a, b).

The hip is dislocated using a spoon-like lever that is placed between the femoral head and the acetabulum. With the hip dislocated, the resection level on the neck can be identified more clearly. The leg is placed slightly across the contralateral one. Resection of the femoral head is performed about 5 mm medial to the intertrochanteric line and at an angle of 50° to the femoral axis. This resection leaves the femoral neck somewhat longer than with standard stems. Only in very contract cases, the femoral neck is osteotomised in situ, and the head is then extracted using a corkscrew-like extractor (Fig. 13.5).

Acetabular Preparation

The acetabulum is now exposed using a bifurcate Hohmann retractor which is placed dorsal and distal to the acetabulum and a pointed wide-bladed curved Hohmann retractor, which is again placed over the anterior acetabular rim.

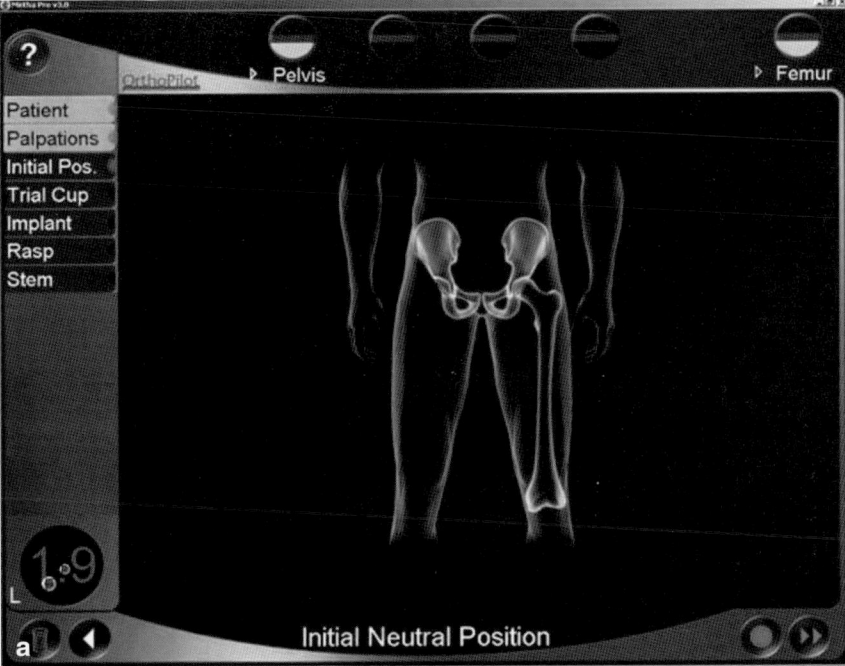

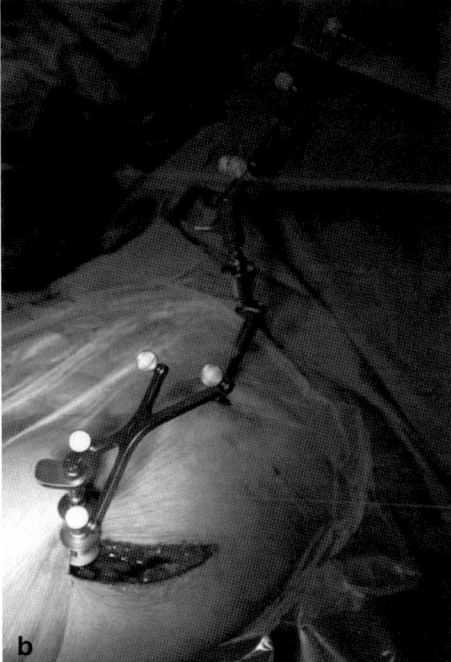

Fig. 13.4 (**a**) Navigation screen for measurement of the initial neutral position. (**b**) Before dislocating the hip, the neutral position is registered with both rigid bodies attached. To go on with surgery, the rigid bodies can be removed temporarily

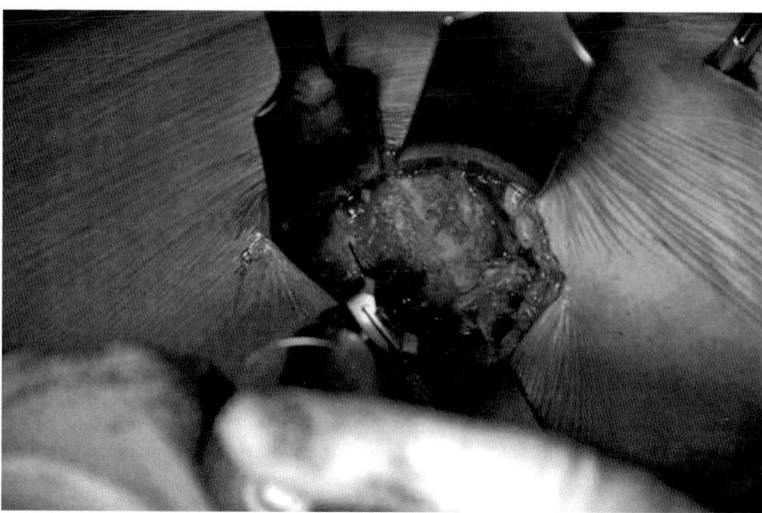

Fig. 13.5 The hip is dislocated to identify the line of resection more clearly, which should be in a 50° angle to the axis of the femur and about 5 mm medial to the trochanter-neck intersection

Occasionally the capsule needs to be retracted which can be done by sutures. The deepest point on the medial wall of the acetabulum is then palpated and recorded using a pointer so that the navigation system can provide information on the depth of reaming and on medial or lateral displacement of the centre of rotation in relation to the original hip centre. The inclination and anteversion of the acetabulum is registered by a trial cup of approximately the diameter of the final cup. This information is displayed on the navigation screen.

Reaming usually starts with a reamer one size smaller than the trial cup. The display of the navigation system provides information on which direction to ream, based on the inclination and anteversion and on the depth relative to the point of the medial wall palpated prior to reaming. Additional information is given about changes of the centre of rotation towards a proximal/distal, medial/lateral and anterior/posterior direction. This helps to influence the final cup position when dysplastic or other deforming conditions have to be corrected. When a good position is achieved and the whole acetabular surface is freed of cartilage and the cortical bone is roughened, so that fine bleeding is visible, the position is recorded (Fig. 13.6a, b).

The acetabular implant is placed and impacted with the navigation system giving information on its position relative to the acetabulum. Our aim is to place the cup at 45° inclination and 15° anteversion, based on the data given by Lewinnek et al. [8] for a "safe zone". When press fit of the implant is achieved in the desired position, the ceramic inlay is inserted and impacted, and the new centre of rotation is recorded with a ball-headed device the size of the chosen head (Fig. 13.7a, b).

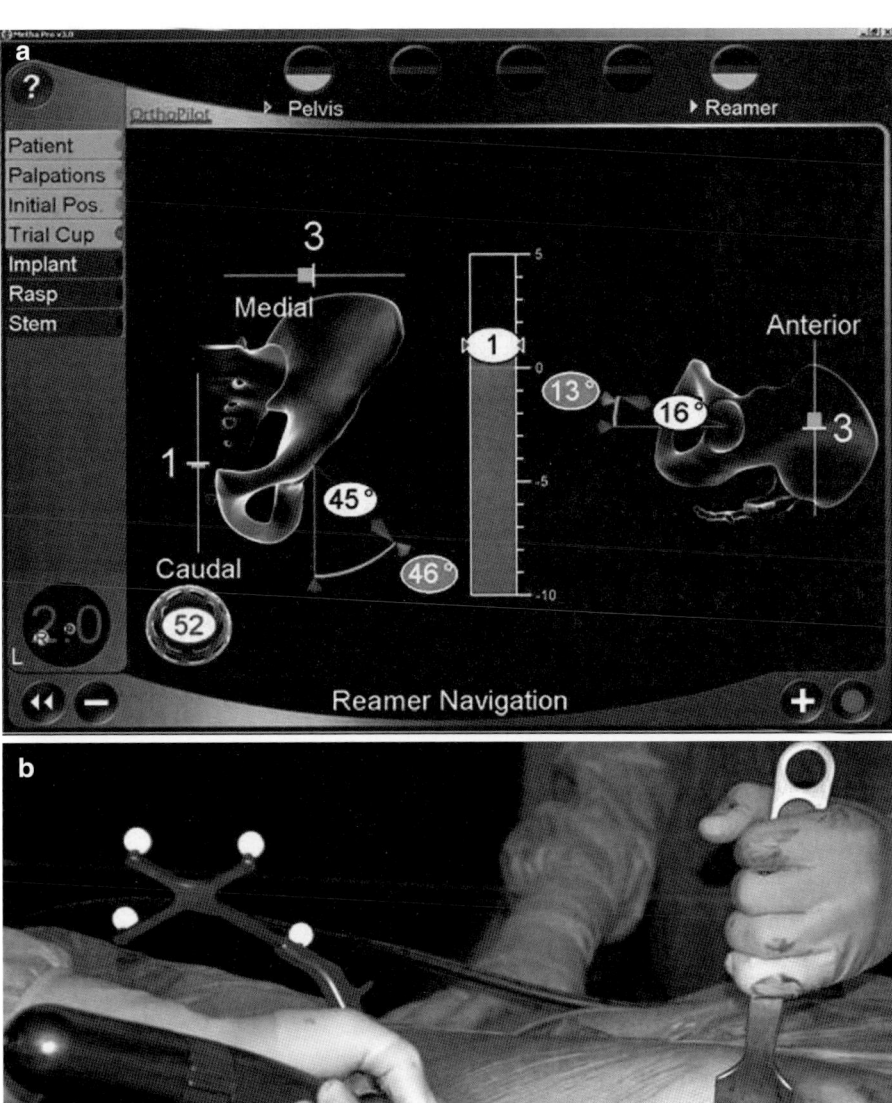

Fig. 13.6 (**a**) Navigation screen for reamer navigation. (**b**) The navigation system provides information on the direction and depth of reaming

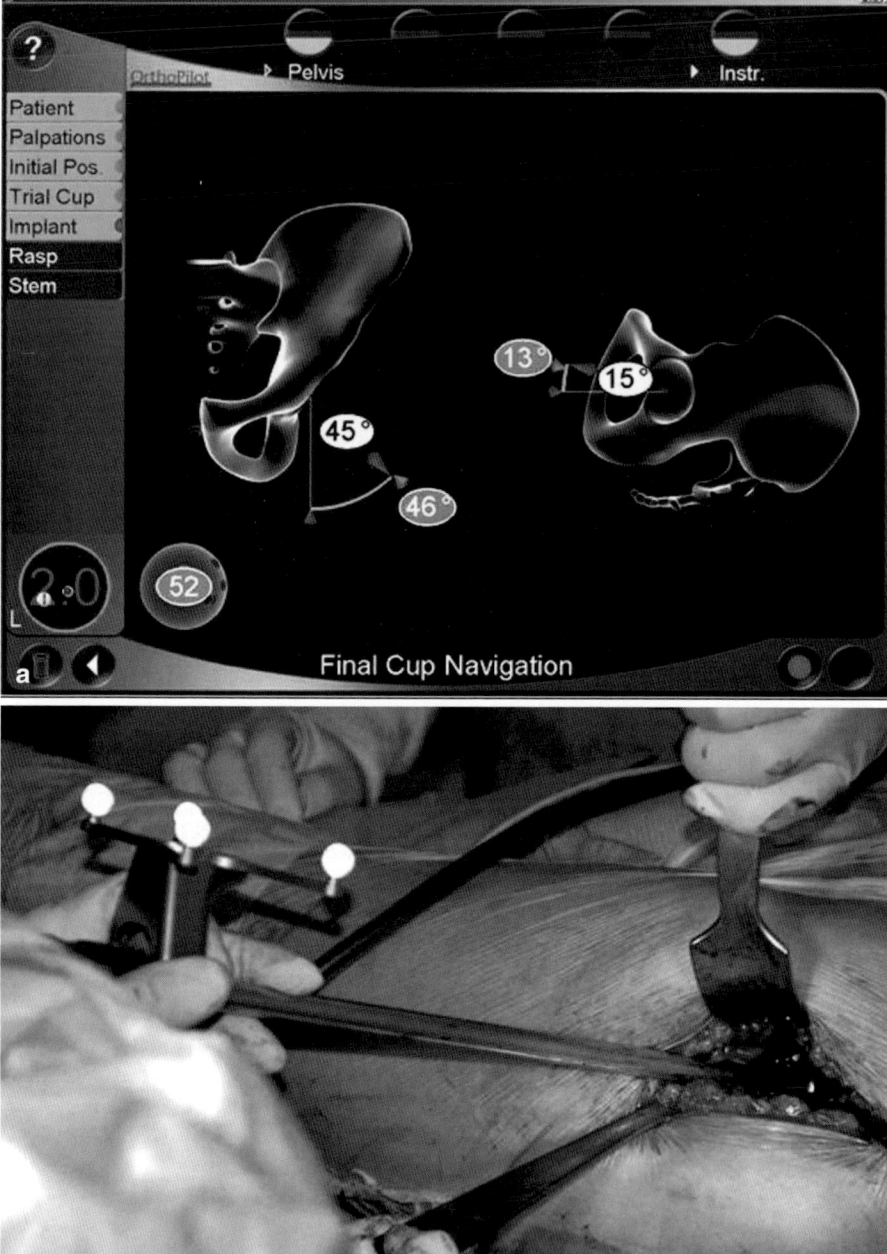

Fig. 13.7 (**a**) Navigation screen for navigating the cup. The navigation system provides information on the direction and depth of reaming. (**b**) The final cup position can be controlled on the screen of the navigation system

Femoral Preparation

The leg is now placed in a 90° external rotation and maximum adduction. The bifurcate Hohmann retractor is placed under the greater trochanter in order to lever it above the iliotibial band, and another more curved bifurcate retractor is placed behind the posterior aspect of medial femoral neck. The resection plane is now visible in its complete circumference. The femoral preparation starts with a bent awl. The point of insertion of the awl is close to the centre of to the neck, first directed towards the lateral femoral cortex and then along the diaphysis. Care has to be taken to prevent perforation of the femoral cortex. A second awl, slightly thicker than the first, is introduced in the same manner. The awls already follow the antetorsion of the femoral neck.

The main idea behind metaphyseal fixation of a short-stemmed prosthesis is that it will be fixed at several points, predetermined by the original anatomy of the femoral neck, metaphysis and proximal diaphysis. These points are not defined in detail and are influenced by the height of the neck resection. It seems essential that cortical contact is achieved at the medial aspect of the neck (calcar femoris), at the anterior and posterior wall and at the lateral edge of the resection plane, about 5 mm medial to the intertrochanteric line. The tip of the prosthesis should also have cortical contact on the lateral and slightly posterior part of the proximal diaphysis. This position can only be influenced to a small degree by voluntarily rotating the awl or the rasps.

The rasps are inserted sequentially. The upper border of the rasp should never dive under the lateral border of the resection level, as this may lead to subsidence of the stem later on. The right position is achieved when no more cancellous bone remains between the rasp and the points mentioned above (Fig. 13.8).

We still prefer a trial reduction to evaluate biomechanics and to have an intra-operative X-ray control in two planes; also the final biomechanics can be simulated. We reduce the hip using a trial neck adapter with a CCD angle of 135° and neutral antetorsion and a medium-size femoral head. We then check for leg length and stability in extended external rotation and in internal rotation in 90° of flexion. With the image intensifier, we take a.p. and frog-leg views. A fissure, fracture or perforation of the femur can be detected; cup positioning and changes in offset or leg length can be evaluated. After redislocation, the rasp is removed and the final implant is inserted and impacted until press-fit fixation is achieved (Fig. 13.9a, b).

Simulation of Biomechanics

The rigid body is secured on the C-clamp and the final position of the implant is recorded. On the navigation screen, the implant size and the head diameter are

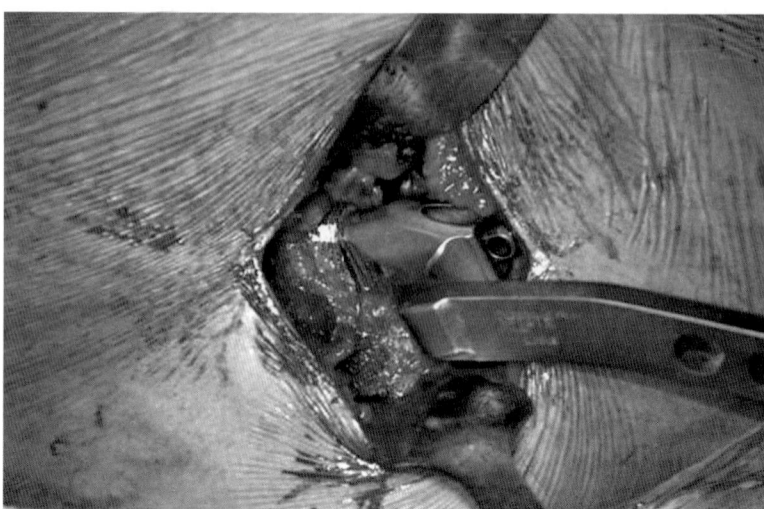

Fig. 13.8 The rasps are inserted sequentially. The right size and position is achieved, when the medial cortex is free of spongious bone and the rasp still leans on the lateral cortex

selected. Now the screen displays the free range of motion possible without dislocation or impingement, the offset changes and the length changes according to the chosen modular neck and head. The data can be changed until the best combination of modular neck cone and head length is identified. By pointing at the screen with a pointing device, the CCD angle can be changed from 130° to 135° and 140°, antetorsion can be changed from −7.5° to neutral to +7.5°, and the head length can be varied from short to XL. We aim for a restoration of offset and a reduction of antetorsion, which is often increased preoperatively. Leg length should be adjusted to the contralateral side. This is often a problem as the methods for preoperative measurement for leg length are mostly not precise enough. For the functional parameters, we aim at an internal rotation in flexion of at least 30° and external rotation in extension of at least 60°; the free flexion angle should exceed 110° without impingement. The chosen modular neck is then inserted and impacted taking great care that the femoral side as well as the neck adapter is meticulously clean and dry, and then the femoral head is placed on the cleansed and dry neck and impacted (Figs. 13.10 and 13.11).

Wound Closure

After reduction of the hip, the flaps of the capsule are sutured in order to try to restore as much of the capsule as possible. A deep suction drain is placed and some light sutures adapt the bluntly split muscles. The iliotibial band is closed with strong sutures, and the wound is finally closed.

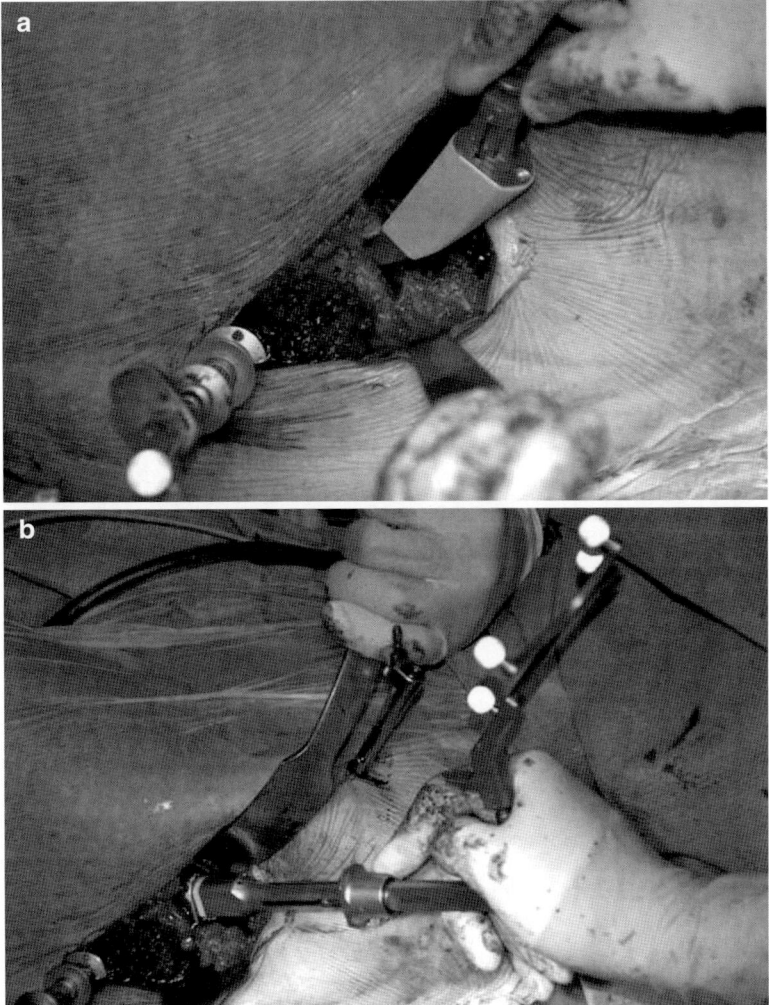

Fig. 13.9 (**a**, **b**) The final implant is inserted and impacted, and then the position is registered for the simulation of biomechanics to choose the optimal modular neck

Aftertreatment

Standard treatment includes a single-shot preoperative antibiotic prophylaxis with cefazolin 2 g and a perioperative thromboprophylaxis with low molecular weight heparin. On the first day after surgery, the patients are mobilised on crutches with full weight bearing. They are told not to adduct or rotate their hips externally for 6 weeks and to use crutches during this period.

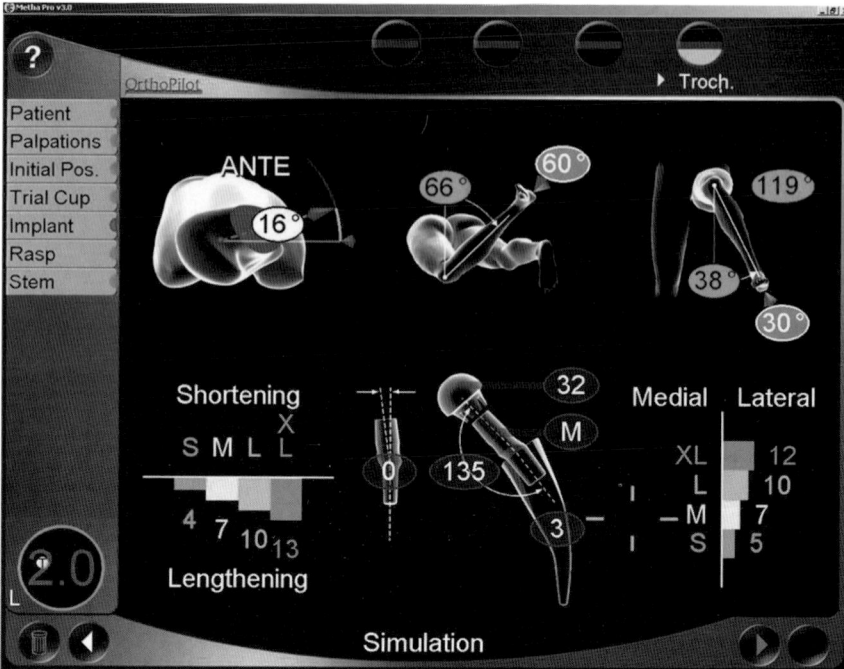

Fig. 13.10 The simulation screen of the navigation gives information on the mechanical changes influenced by the choice of the modular neck. In the centre, the antetorsion (here 0°) and the CCD angle (here: 135°) can be varied. The effect can be seen on the three pictures above: the antetorsion, the safe ROM for external rotation of the extended leg, and the safe ROM for internal rotation for the hip flexed at 90°. It is also influenced by the head size. The offset and leg lengthening changes are displayed for all different head neck lengths

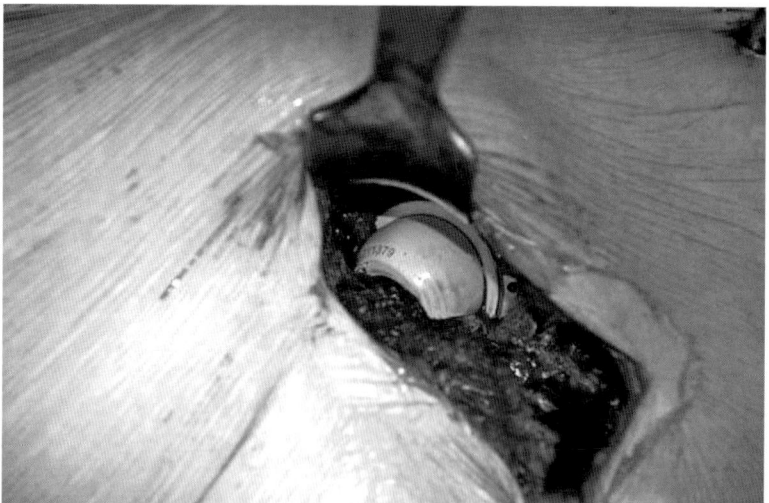

Fig. 13.11 Final reposition of the hip with all components in place

Results

One intraoperative perforation of the lateral cortical bone occurred when the first rasp was inserted, but this had no influence on the course of surgery or the clinical outcome. The average duration of surgery was 67 min. Average intraoperative blood loss was 350 ml.

Cup

In group 1 (cup navigation only), the average cup position was 45.6° of inclination and 15.9° of anteversion and in group 2 (cup and stem navigation) 45.2° and 17.3°, respectively. The centre of rotation was changed to 1.1 mm lateral, 0.6 mm distal and 0.6 mm posterior in group 1 and 1.2 mm medial, 0.1 mm distal and 1.4 mm anterior in group 2. The mean cup size was 50 mm in group 1 and 52 mm in group 2.

Stem and Modular Neck

In group 1 (cup navigation only), the modular neck adapter used most frequently was 135° (standard) ($n = 27$) with neutral antetorsion or −7.5° retroversion (−7.5° $n = 13$, 0° $n = 14$); the 130° neck adapter was used in 21 cases. In group 2 (fully navigated), neck adapters of all CCD angles were used. The neck adapter use most often had −7.5° of retroversion and in few cases neutral or anteverted (−7.5° $n = 120$, 0° $n = 75$, +7.5° $n = 15$). The average antetorsion of the stem was 20.4°, with a range of −5.3° to 56.6°, so that the overall antetorsion remained positive in all cases except of one (Fig. 13.12a, b).

The length of the ceramic heads were 25 short, 20 medium, 14 long and 1 extra long head in group 1 and 55 short, 114 medium, 39 long and 2 extra long heads in group 2.

Only for the fully navigated group 2 reliable leg length and offset measurements could be recorded by the navigation system. The mean lengthening in group 2 was 8.3 mm for the stem and 6.1 mm overall, and for offset 1.0 mm of medialisation for the stem and 4.6 mm of medialisation overall. The size distribution of the stems can be seen in Table 13.1.

Radiological Results

In four cases, the distal tip of the prosthesis did not reach the lateral cortex and the prosthesis was placed in valgus. The position did not change in the follow-up radiographs. Two cases of subsidence, 3 and 4 mm, respectively, occurred, both

Fig. 13.12 (**a, b**) Distribution
of the modular necks for
group 1 (**a**), where only the
cup was navigated, and group
2 (**b**) with cup and stem
navigation and simulation of
the biomechanics. Group 2
shows more variability

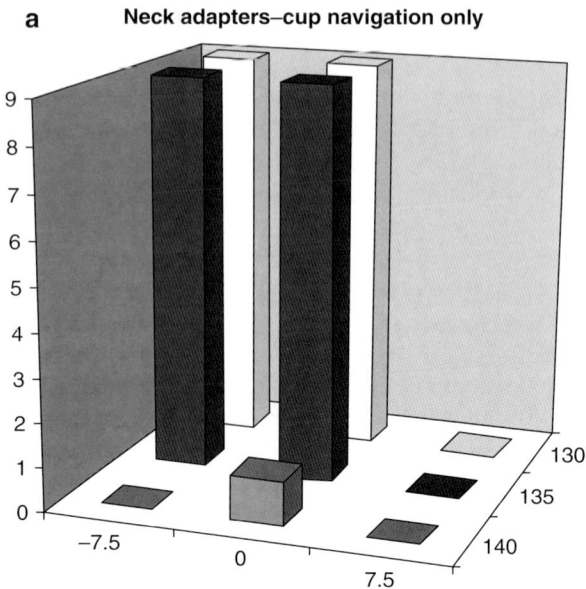

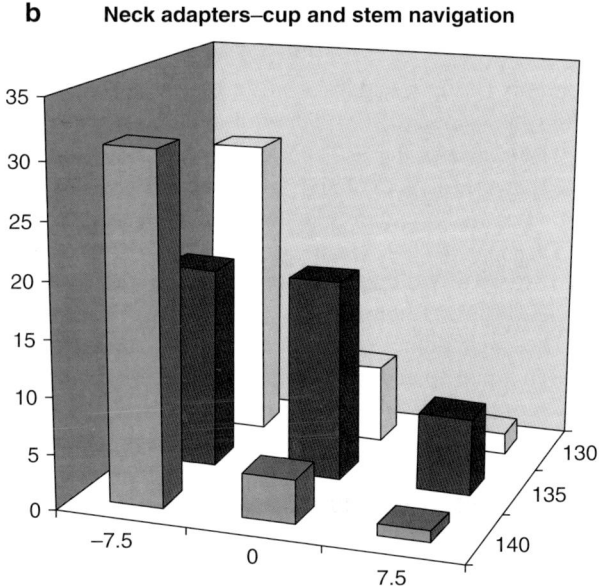

without clinical complaints. We assume that the chosen stem had been undersized
intraoperatively. On the axial view of the radiographic controls, there seemed to be
still some cancellous bone between the prosthesis and the cortical bone of the neck.
Six months postoperatively, the subsidence stopped and the implant has remained
stable, without any clinical symptoms. While these stems probably were undersized,
we had three cases of fissuring of the femoral neck, two of which were stabilised
with a cerclage. We think these cases are due to our learning curve while finding the

Table 13.1 Distribution of stem sizes

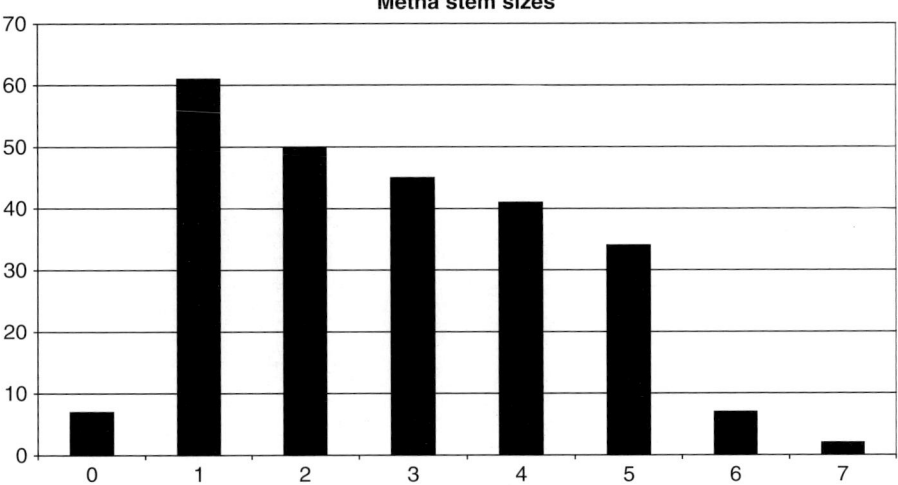

right implant position and size. All these cases occurred in the first year. Only one radiolucent line was found in a prosthesis implanted recently, which is suspicious of a deep infection and is under investigation at the moment (Fig. 13.13).

Clinical Results

Lengthening up to 3.5 cm was possible. No dislocation occurred. No thrombosis or vascular lesion was observed. There was only one superficial wound infection and one temporary femoral nerve palsy. Patients reported a faster postoperative recovery with earlier stability and earlier stair climbing. Although we were not able to collect more detailed data on this, our physiotherapists support this clinical impression (Tables 13.2 and 13.3).

Conclusion and Discussion

Our reason to change from a good functioning standard hip system to a short modular stem prosthesis was to improve further on long-term and short-term outcomes. We cannot judge on the long-term outcomes at this time. Still the theoretical advantages are promising. We had less bone loss and the prosthesis does not affect the diaphysis, also leaving the modulus of elasticity unchanged. The neck is cut higher compared to straight stem prosthesis, and the greater trochanter region is left untouched. In addition, the metaphysis is not filled up but leaves spongious bone, while the prosthesis secures contact with the cortical bone at different points. This all should lead to better bone stock in case of revision.

Fig. 13.13 Postoperative
X-ray of a Metha prosthesis
with 36 mm head

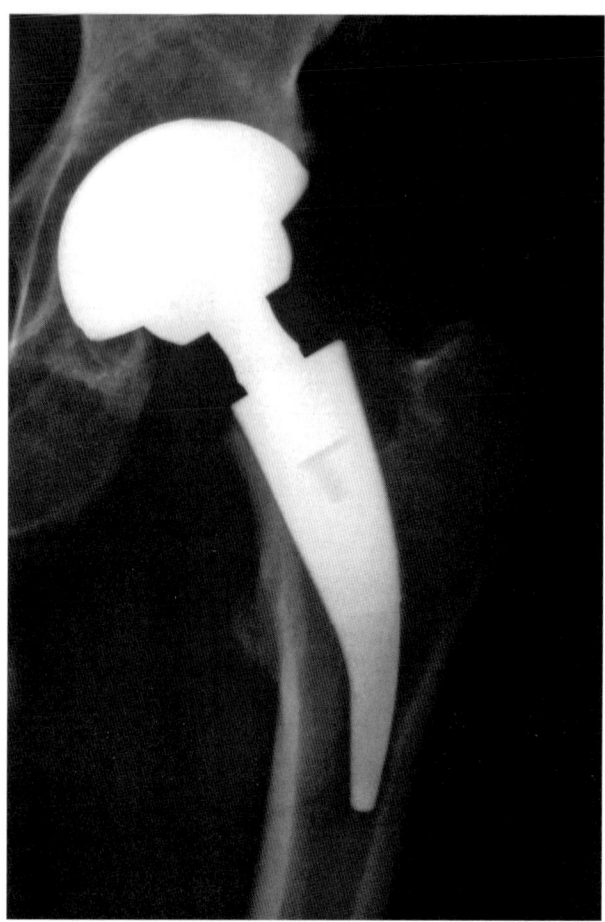

Table 13.2 Femoral head sizes and length

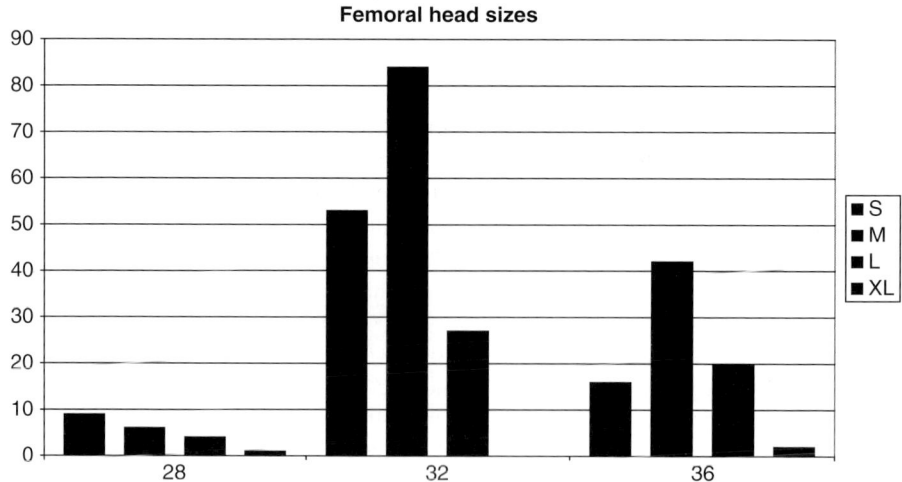

Table 13.3 Offset changes and lengthening of the femur

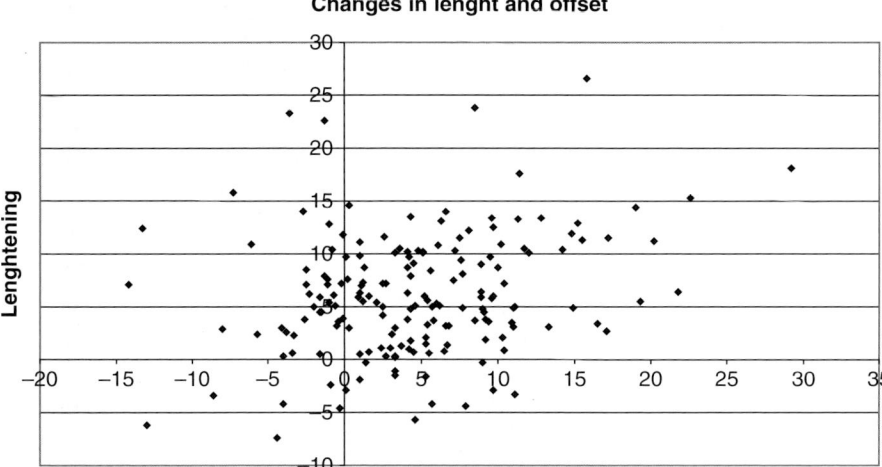

The suitability of the short-stemmed prosthesis for a less invasive procedure could be confirmed in this series. Using a modified Watson-Jones approach, detachment of muscles was not necessary, and it was not affected by the need for placing the rigid bodies necessary for navigation. The femoral C-clamp could be positioned through this approach. The screw on the iliac crest required another incision but gave more stability than a Steinmann nail, which can be inserted through the main incision. Yet the procedure could be done using incisions of 8–10 cm.

Good primary stability could be achieved. Only two stems subsided, which is due to our learning curve, as well as the early fissures. In subsequent cases, these problems have not occurred. Still the choice of the right size, which cannot be determined exactly by preoperative radiographs, remains one of the main issues.

Modularity should lead to a better restoration of biomechanics [6]. We evaluated the modularity with respect to the hip geometry. In group 1 without navigation the surgeons tended to use a neutral antetorsion and midsize CCD angle. In the navigation group, a more differentiated choice with more retroversion and varus necks. We think it is due to the patient selection with a high percentage of dysplastic hips, where the increased antetorsion and valgus of the neck had to be corrected.

With a wide range of different neck and head sizes, however, the overall leg length still could not be adjusted in all cases. In our opinion, more different modular necks would be beneficial to correct the pre-existing deformities towards average hip biomechanics.

Navigation is considered to increase the accuracy of positioning in total hip arthroplasty [9]. Its reliability has been proven for the acetabulum and for the femoral stem [4, 10]. While the aim for the placement of the acetabulum is clear, the parameters for the stem differ. For the cup, the centre of rotation should be undisplaced, and the values for inclination and anteversion should be in the range described by Lewinnek et al. [8].

In modular short-stemmed prosthesis, the placement of the stem only takes care of maximal stability in the femoral metaphysis. Fixation of the stem is independent from restoration of biomechanics of the hip through the choice of the modular neck. Navigation therefore differs from that in standard hips. The stem itself is not navigated, but the choice of the optimal modular neck and head and joint reconstruction is. The criteria for restoration are offset, leg length antetorsion, centre of rotation of the head and range of motion of the implant. These parameters can be controlled using navigation. By calculating the safe range of motion and the maximum flexion without impingement, the navigation system was able to help to find the right biomechanics independent from the changes in the geometry of the hips. No dislocation was seen in the intraoperative test as well as in the postoperative follow-up.

In our experience, the navigated short-stemmed prosthesis offered good intraoperative handling and good short-term results.

Acknowledgements The authors did not receive any outside funding or grants in support of their research for or preparation of this work. Neither they nor a member of their immediate families received payments or other benefits or a commitment or agreement to provide such benefits from a commercial entity. No commercial entity paid or directed, or agreed to pay or direct, any benefits to a research fund, foundation, division, centre, clinical practice, or other charitable nonprofit organisation with which the authors, or a member of their immediate families, are affiliated or associated.

The authors declare that the work described in this chapter complies with current laws of the country in which it was performed.

References

1. Morrey BF, Adams RA, Kessler M (2000) A conservative femoral replacement for total hip arthroplasty. A prospective study. J Bone Joint Surg Br 82(7):952–958
2. Sculco TP (2004) Minimally invasive total hip arthroplasty: in the affirmative. J Arthroplasty 19(4 Suppl 1):78–80
3. Hube R, Zage M, Hein W, Reichel H (2004) Frühfunktionelle Ergebnisse einer Kurzschaftprothese des Hüftgelenks mit metaphysär-intertrochantärer Verankerung [Early functional results with the Mayo-hip, a short stem system with metaphyseal-intertrochanteric fixation]. Orthopädie 33:1249–1258
4. Lazovic D, Kaib N (2005) Results with navigated bicontact total hip arthroplasty. Orthopedics 28(10 Suppl):s1227–s1233
5. Lazovic D, Zigan R (2006) Navigation of short-stem implants. Orthopedics 29(10 Suppl):S125–S129
6. Chmell MJ, Rispler D, Poss R (1995) The impact of modularity in total hip arthroplasty. Clin Orthop Relat Res 319:77–84
7. Watson-Jones R (1936) Fractures of the neck of the femur. Br J Surg 23:787–808
8. Lewinnek GE, Lewis JL, Tarr R, Compere CL, Zimmerman JR (1978) Dislocations after total hip-replacement arthroplasties. J Bone Joint Surg Am 60(2):217–220
9. DiGioia AM, Jaramaz B, Blackwell M, Simon DA, Morgan F, Moody JE, Nikou C, Colgan BD, Aston CA, Labarca RS, Kischell E, Kanade T (1998) Image guided navigation system to measure intraoperatively acetabular implant alignment. Clin Orthop Relat Res 355:8–22
10. Kiefer H, Othman A (2005) OrthoPilot total hip arthroplasty workflow and surgery. Orthopedics 28(10 Suppl):s1221–s1226

Printing: Ten Brink, Meppel, The Netherlands
Binding: Stürtz, Würzburg, Germany